An MD is Not Enough

How to Survive and Thrive in Medicine

Kimberly Kinder, MD

Copyright © 2019 Kimberly Kinder
All rights reserved.
ISBN-13: 9781086461183

This book is dedicated to my husband, Jesse. Thank you for your love and support in everything I do!

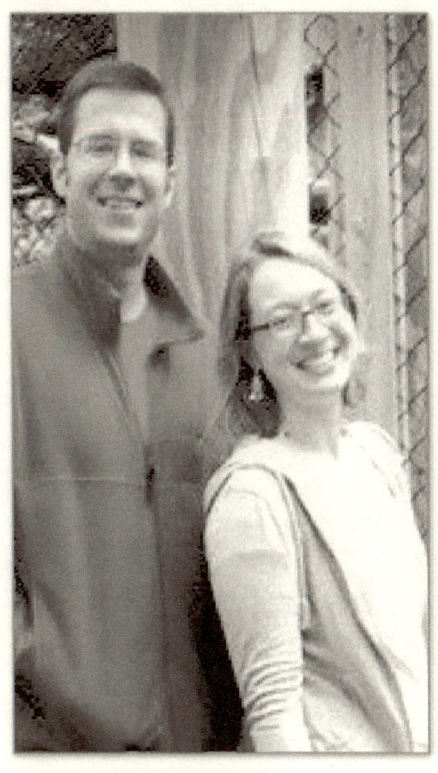

Table of Contents

Introduction	1
SECTION ONE: Choosing Your Path	3
Chapter One: Medical School Selection	4
Chapter Two: Specialty Selection	9
Chapter Three: Residency Selection	24
Chapter Four: Residency Application	31
Chapter Five: Choices During Residency	40
Chapter Six: Choosing Your Career	43
SECTION TWO: Getting the Job	51
Chapter One: Preparing Your Application	52
Chapter Two: Applying for Jobs	59
Chapter Three: The Job Interview	64
Chapter Four: Contracts	68
SECTION THREE: Doing the Job	83
Chapter One: Taking Care of Yourself	84
Chapter Two: Scheduling	91
Chapter Three: Electronic Medical Record	94
Chapter Four: Medical Coding	98
SECTION FOUR: Financial (and Life) Planning	131
Chapter One: Life Planning	132
Chapter Two: Insurance	143
Chapter Three: Financial Planning	150
Conclusion	164
Appendix 1: Website Links	165
Appendix 2: Additional books you might find helpful	169
Appendix 3: EMR help	171

Introduction

When I told my physicist husband that I wanted to write a book and what it was about, he mentioned a book that he had found helpful in his career. It was called *A PhD is Not Enough* and was written by physicist Peter J. Feibelman. I kind of ignored my husband — I wasn't trying to get a PhD, after all — and ended up writing *Communication in Medicine: A guide for students and physicians on interacting with patients, colleagues, and everyone else.*

While writing *Communication in Medicine*, I often thought of additional information I wished I had known earlier in my career. I kept coming up with more and more subjects: Where should I do my residency? What can I expect in a physician contract? How in the world do I code patient encounters? I decided that I wanted to write a second book that covered these topics and more. I realized that the current book is much more along the lines of *A PhD is Not Enough*, but for the medical profession, so I named it with the inspiration of Dr. Feibelman's text. (It's usually good to listen to your spouse, too.)

This book is not a substitute for the financial planners, lawyers, medical coders, and other professionals who make a living with their knowledge of these topics. Instead, it gives you the information you need to know to get you started in each field. It is better to understand some basic contract terminology before you talk to a lawyer so you're not spending $300 per hour learning about it. You want to know a little about the type of investment opportunities available before you trust your hard-earned money to a financial planner.

My information comes from residency lectures, discussions with colleagues, working with some of these professionals, reading literature on the topics, and personal experience. I try to use real examples whenever possible, so ENT (ear/nose/throat) will be mentioned more than other specialties in certain sections since that is the field where I have the most firsthand knowledge. Even though ENT is mentioned frequently, the information applies to all specialties. Since this is an amalgamation, I do not have true "references." However, I have provided a list of websites and books at the end that I have found helpful, and have mentioned some of them in the text where appropriate.

This book is arranged in four sections that are semi-chronological. For example, you need to choose your residency before you go out and get a job. You will want to work on managing finances throughout your life, though, not just once you complete residency. I recommend reading the entire book in order and then referring back to sections as they again become relevant throughout your career.

You clearly need a strong medical fund of knowledge and patient care skills to be a successful physician. These things are what medical school and residency will likely provide. However, an understanding of the complementary issues covered here will help your life and career run more smoothly. I have tried my best to share as much information as possible, so I hope you enjoy reading this book. I also hope that having this information makes a lot of these processes less stressful for you than they (at times) have been for me!

SECTION ONE: Choosing Your Path

You will make many choices in your career as a physician. Some days during residency, I felt like I had to make so many decisions that when I went home and my husband asked what I wanted to watch on TV, I was so "decisioned-out" that I had to make him choose. You will be bombarded with numerous daily decisions, many of which put patient lives on the line. Your training will hopefully teach you how to deal with these types of decisions. This section, though, deals with the long-lasting decisions you make for yourself in your medical career.

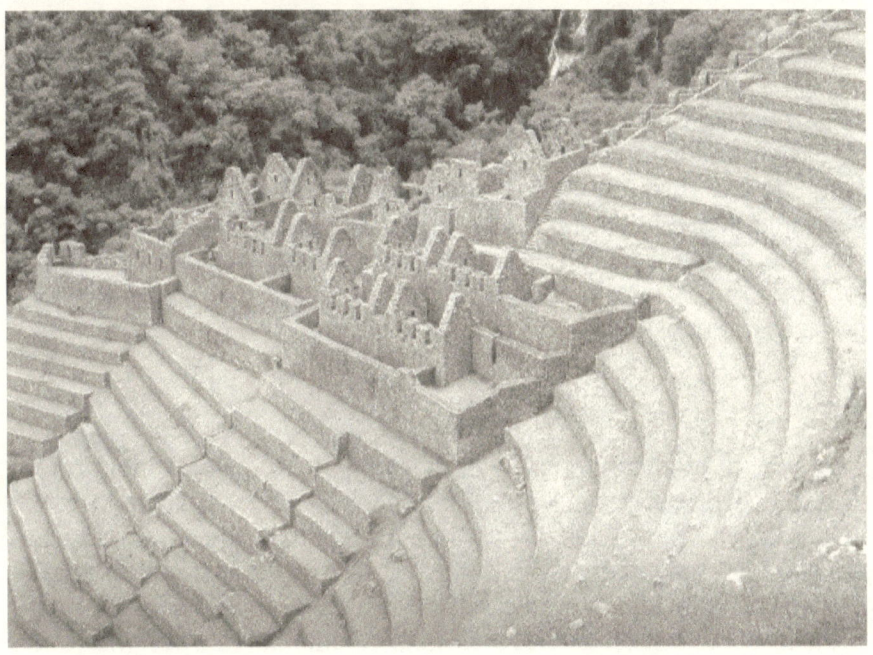

A portion of Wiñay Wayna ruins along the Inca Trail
One of the great "paths" of history...

Chapter One: Medical School Selection

You may have already done this part, but this section may still be helpful background information when you are applying for residencies or jobs. According to Wikipedia, there are 141 allopathic (MD) medical schools and 31 osteopathic (DO) schools in the US. This is much more limited than the over 4000 undergraduate universities listed by Wikipedia, but still gives you a lot of choices. I have included a couple websites in the index that have a comprehensive listing of schools if you want to start from scratch, but most people will want to shorten the list with some of the factors listed below.

1. Geographic Location

This may limit your choice of medical school for several reasons. You likely have some idea of where you want to live — big city vs. small town, east coast vs. west coast, warm weather vs. four seasons. If you have a spouse, his or her job or education may be tied to a certain location. You may want to stay close to your family for support, especially if you are raising your own children while going to medical school.

2. Cost

The cost of medical school varies widely, with tuition ranging from free to over $50,000 per year. Some schools offer significantly lower tuition for in-state residents, so this may tie in to the location factor, as well. You may consider looking into state residency requirements if a school you are interested in offers an in-state discount. If you want to do research or need to take additional courses (i.e. post-baccalaureate training) prior to starting medical school, it might be advantageous to do it in the state where you plan to go to obtain your professional degree. Some of the websites in the index give you access to published tuition rates.

3. Size

Medical school class sizes vary. I interviewed at four schools, with a range of class size from about 100 to 250. Most medical schools do large lectures, smaller lab classes, and group learning. Because of this, I do not see the overall class size as a very important number, but you want to find out how the teaching is done ahead of time. If you are sitting in a nephrology lecture, it does not really matter if there are 20 students or 200 students. However, you want to make sure there are enough instructors in your histology and anatomy labs so you can ask questions when needed. I shared my gross anatomy cadaver with 3 other students, which seemed reasonable. Cadavers can be hard to acquire, so you may want to check on this at your prospective school.

4. Ranking or "Prestige"

U.S. News & World Report (link in index) provides annual rankings of medical schools for both research and primary care. This is overrated in some ways, since almost anyone who graduates from an accredited US medical school will be able to match into a residency and then practice medicine. However, if you are applying for a highly competitive residency (e.g. dermatology, ENT, neurosurgery), it is often helpful to go to a highly ranked medical school. The medical school ranking these residencies are usually looking at is the *U.S. News* research ranking. Your medical school will be forever listed on your CV, so a more prestigious medical school may help you in future job searches, as well. Therefore, if you can get into one of these schools and it seems like a good fit for you, you may want to strongly consider it. You need to be realistic about the strength of your application, though. If you did not get great test scores or do research, you may not get into the "top" schools.

5. Specialty

This partially ties into the previous factor. If you already know what type of doctor you want to be, you may want to go to a medical school that places many graduates into that specialty. If you want to do research or primary care, you can start with *U.S. News*. If your interests lie elsewhere, you may want to look directly at the medical school's website. Medical schools keep records of their graduates. If the match information is not published on their website, you can always ask the admissions people at the school. However, many people who enter medical school with one specialty in mind end up choosing a different field during the four years of school. It is important to obtain a well-rounded education as you might decide you love a specialty that you had never previously considered.

6. Allopathic vs. Osteopathic

The vast majority of physicians in the US choose to go to an allopathic (MD) medical school. This is the more traditional path, and prepares you to go into any field. Osteopathic (DO) programs are less common and have a slightly different focus. Students still obtain most of the same information as in an MD program, but also take a more "holistic approach" to healing. Osteopathic programs include instruction in physical manipulation techniques, as well. Admission rates are often higher at osteopathic schools. Most residency programs will accept both MD and DO applicants, but DO applicants are sometimes seen as less competitive by residency review committees. Although this is the traditional model and bias, it does not always hold true. I recently spoke to an undergraduate who was applying to medical schools. He said an MD program he spoke to talked about how "well-rounded" it wanted its students to be, while the DO program was "focused on strong academics."

7. Fit

This is the least scientific but potentially the most important factor. You cannot fully assess this issue until you visit the school and meet the people, though, so you will want to choose where to apply based on the above factors (and any others that might be important to you). When interviewing at each school, you need to listen to your instincts to try to figure out if you will be happy at that particular place. I had the whole spectrum of positive impressions, neutral impressions, and negative impressions from the schools I visited. I looked at the school websites and talked to people before I visited, but this often contradicted the actual feel I had during the interview. You're going to spend a lot of time with these people, so you want to feel as comfortable as possible.

8. Curriculum structure

The traditional structure of medical school is 2 years of classroom work followed by 2 years of clinical experience. Classroom work usually includes basic anatomy, pathology, histology, and pharmacology. Mine had some of this basic information first, followed by "organ system blocks" that incorporated more detail on each of these topics. There will be both lectures and lab sections. Group learning is becoming more and more prevalent. If lecture vs. group learning matters to you, make sure you find out the structure of the preclinical years at your prospective medical school. Many medical schools are trying to provide earlier exposure to patients, as well. My school had 18 months of classroom work, and then we started on our core clerkships. The core clerkships are a year-long set of rotations that all students complete. There are some slight variations on exactly what is included, but all schools will cover the "basics" of surgery, internal medicine, pediatrics, family medicine, and OB. The rest of medical school (12 to 18 months depending on your program) is devoted to electives, upperclass seminars, and sometimes research. I don't think that early exposure to patients is a critical factor, but it was nice to complete my core clerkships early to have more elective time. You'll have the rest of your life to see patients! However, if you're debating between 2 programs you like, this may help you choose.

Another thing to consider with 'curriculum structure' is pursuing an MD-PhD program. You generally apply to this program when applying to medical school, but there may be limited options to join a program partway through medical school. This usually takes 7-9 years to complete (rather than the 4 for medical school), but you earn both your MD and PhD during the process. MD-PhD programs often cover tuition and provide a stipend, as well. If you have a strong interest in research, this may be a good option. However, if you are just doing it for "free medical school," it is probably not the best financial decision. By spending more time in school, you are delaying your time to start as an attending. That's when you make real money. So although you aren't getting into as much debt, it may not be financially beneficial in the long run. Also, there is a big difference between medical school and graduate school. Every day that I showed up and did what I was supposed to do as a medical student, I was 1 day closer to earning my degree. My husband – who was in graduate school for physics – had to hope that his experiments would work, the journal referees would choose to accept his papers, and the thesis committee would approve of his overall body of work. Just showing up does not lead to a PhD.

Chapter Two: Specialty Selection

Ever since you can remember, you've wanted to be a pediatric hematologist. But why is that? Is that really the "right" field for you, or did you happen to meet a pediatric hematologist who inspired you so much that you wanted to be just like him? Strong mentors can make a lasting impression, but you have to try to assess what *your* career would be like in that specialty rather than what *that person* has done. If you have a specialty in mind, it is fine to work toward that. You definitely want to keep an open mind, though, because you might find something that you love even more than your original choice.

Many resources are available to help you choose a specialty, in addition to using the information I present here. One of the most important things is talking to physicians practicing in specialties that interest you. Specific discussion topics are referenced below, and you may want to ask them generally what they like and dislike about the field, how they got into it, and how to pursue your interest in that field. Numerous websites can help you choose your specialty, as well, and I have listed some in the index. The problem that I find is that most publications by official organizations have to try to be politically correct. I have no organizational affiliation, so while I try to avoid being derogatory toward any field, I am not limited like some of the websites.

1. First Decision: Medicine vs. Surgery

Most people will tell you that you first want to decide if you are going to choose a medical or a surgical field. Generally, if you like to think through solutions to problems, you choose medicine, and if you like to use your hands or physically fix things, you choose surgery. This is partially true, but there are some flaws to this logic. First, there are many specialties that do not fit into medicine vs. surgery. Second, there are a number in fields of medicine that are quite procedure-heavy, such as interventional cardiology. Third, some surgical specialties (like ENT, for example) do not have a medical counterpart, so you end up providing both surgical and medical care. Although medicine vs. surgery can be a good start, we will soon review some of the factors that can help you actually choose which specialty is right for you.

2. Second Decision: The Actual Specialty

For some specialties, you don't actually have to decide on your specialty until it comes time to do a fellowship. Most internal medicine and pediatric subspecialties require you to do a 3-year residency and then a 2-3 year fellowship. If you are trying to choose among nephrology, medical genetics, and endocrinology, you won't have to do so until you are already partway through your residency. General surgery also has multiple fellowships if you want to subspecialize after the 5-year general surgery residency. Some specialties can be accessed through multiple pathways. For example, you can become a sports medicine specialist by starting with an emergency medicine, family medicine, or pediatrics residency. Outside of the paths discussed above, you apply for most specialties right out of medical school. There is a link in the index of all of the residencies and fellowships that participate in ERAS (Electronic Residency Application Service), or what is commonly called "The Match." It is important to know that both accredited and non-accredited fellowships also exist outside of ERAS. After completing an ENT residency, you can do a fellowship in neurotology, pediatric ENT, laryngology, facial plastics, head and neck reconstruction, or rhinology — just to name a few.

3. Third Decision: Additional Research Time?

The residency for each specialty has a minimum required length: 3 years for emergency medicine, 4 years for OB/GYN, 6 years for plastic surgery, etc. Many residencies give you an option to add on 1-2 years devoted to research. Research is generally incorporated into traditional residencies, too. For example, in my regular 5-year ENT residency, we had a 4-month research block in the fourth year and an annual resident research day. If the option is available, the decision about whether or not to devote extra time to research in your training is entirely up to you. If you are interested in doing research as part of your career, it makes sense to consider incorporating additional research time into your training. Do NOT do it just because someone tells you you should.

4. Choose What You Love

In your medical school basic science curriculum, you may find that cardiac physiology fascinates you. On your internal medicine rotation, you love reading EKGs. You enjoy forming lasting relationships with patients. It sounds like cardiology is the right field for you. Some people will be lucky and fall in love with a certain field. You just need to make sure it is really the specialty that you love and you are not merely enamored by a mentor in that field. One of the plastic surgeons I worked with in medical school was an amazing person and physician. I knew that I did not really enjoy the types of procedures he did or the attitudes of some of the cosmetic patients, though, so I knew that plastic surgery was not the specialty for me. I had a great time on the rotation, but it was really because of the preceptor and not the field.

5. Choose What You Like

If you don't fall in love, you still need a way to find your ideal specialty. Each specialty has pros and cons, and your day-to-day work can really vary based on which field you choose. There are also factors you will be able to modify with decisions you make when choosing your actual job, which we will discuss in a later chapter. For now, here is a discussion of factors you may want to consider when choosing your specialty.

Patient Age: If you love children, consider general pediatrics or a pediatric subspecialty. If you enjoy working with the elderly, you may want to do a geriatric medicine fellowship after an internal medicine or family medicine residency. Geriatric patients are statistically closer to the ends of their lives, so make sure you are OK with the fact that you'll have to deal with a higher patient mortality rate. If you like all ages, consider family medicine. Some specialties like ENT and emergency medicine will see patients of all ages, as well, but many medical and surgical specialties are broken up into adult vs. pediatric practitioners.

Patient Acuity: Some doctors like to see the sickest patients, while others prefer healthier ones. If you love the adrenaline rush that comes with life-or-death situations and you feel a strong sense of accomplishment from helping someone who is critically ill recover from their disease, you may enjoy emergency medicine, critical care medicine, or trauma surgery. As with advanced patient age, though, these patients have a higher mortality rate. It can be very hard emotionally when patients pass away. If you do better talking to patients in a calm outpatient setting and getting them to change their habits before they get to the life-or-death situation, you might like medicine or one of its subspecialties. Many specialties have a mix of both, and you can tailor your practice to help the types of patients that most appeal to you after finishing your training. Make sure you are honest with yourself. We need doctors to take care of both types of patients. In residency, you will tend to see sicker patients than you will out in practice, unless you intentionally seek them out. I am surprised in my practice by how many patients simply want reassurance that they are OK, or that the lump they noted is not cancer. Even though I may not be "saving lives" in these situations, it is still valuable for the patients to have that peace of mind.

Hospital vs. Outpatient: This partially ties in with the patient acuity issue, as you generally see sicker patients in the hospital and healthier patients in a clinic setting. However, the idea with this topic is really the flow of your work day. In a hospital, you will generally "round" on patients at least once per day, and sometimes much more often. Rounding can be physically examining and speaking with the patient, or discussing the patient with other caregivers. You will make a plan for what you want to accomplish for each patient during the day. This is sometimes quite straightforward, but at other times involves significant critical thinking. You then execute your plan and make revisions as you go. You may be on call for these patients once you leave the hospital, or you may sign-out to another provider. The opposite to this is a pure clinic setting, where patients come to an office to see you, generally with a prearranged schedule for the day. You might spend anywhere from 10 to 60 minutes with a given patient, where you focus exclusively on that patient and try to solve whatever issue is most pressing. You may schedule a follow up visit if needed to assess your intervention. If you really like one of these ways of caring for patients over the other, try to choose a specialty where you are able to do that. Many specialties have options for either model. For example, as a pulmonologist, you could have mostly an outpatient clinic, or you could choose to staff an ICU where you spend your days in the hospital. Most anesthesiologists work in a hospital or surgery center, but those who go on to do a pain management fellowship may run an outpatient clinic instead. Again, if you really like a certain specialty and want to work in a certain setting, talk to people in that specialty to see what they think.

Income: This is probably pretty obvious to you, but income varies widely across specialties. According to the Medscape 2019 Physician Compensation Report (link in index), primary care physicians (PCPs) earned an average of $237,000 and specialists earned an average of $341,000. These are at least 20% higher than the 2015 numbers, so that is good news for doctors. Of the specific fields they surveyed, orthopedic surgeons earned the most ($482,000), while public health physicians earned the least ($209,000). This being said, if you cannot make a living on $209,000, you need to refer to Section Four of this book ASAP. You may hear stories of PCPs being "unable to pay off debt," but I think this is generally much more of a budgeting issue than a true income problem. If you were only making $30,000 a year, that would be a different story, but that is not the case. Having a higher income specialty may allow you to work less (either fewer total years or fewer hours per week) or may make it easier for you to live the lifestyle you desire, but please do not make your specialty decision based on salary alone. If you hate your job, almost no amount of money can make it worth doing. Also, remember that Medscape and other similar resources tend to give averages. You may make far more or far less than the average in your actual job.

"Thinking" vs. "Doing:" Surgeons are not just technicians — we actually do think about our patients and our plan for the operation. However, the time spent in discussing the pharmacokinetics of each class of diabetes medication on my medicine rounds was — let's just say — "less than enjoyable" for me. One of my best friends in medical school loved it, though, and strongly considered becoming an endocrinologist. When learning about the thyroid gland, did you like the hormone production and feedback process or the hands-on anatomy? For me, being able to physically remove the thyroid gland is more fun than calculating the appropriate dose of levothyroxine for a patient. If you like "thinking," medical specialties are often preferable. If you prefer "doing," choose a surgical or other procedure-oriented field.

6. Avoid What You Hate

Hopefully, there are some specialties that appeal to you because of their positive characteristics. However, you want to make sure you don't choose a field that has something you really hate, as this may be enough to outweigh all the positives. One of my senior colleagues in medical school told me that people choose their field based on "what bothers them the least." (He was specifically referring to types of bodily secretions — colorectal surgeons can deal with feces, OB/GYNs can handle vaginal secretions, and ENTs can do snot — but this concept applies equally well to less distasteful subjects.) You can flip to the negative side of the "Choose What You Like" section above to consider some of these topics. Several additional factors are listed below.

Call Responsibility: I would like being a surgeon so much better if I did not have to take call. Call frustrates me because of the limits it puts on my social activities and its interruption of my sleep. It can be infuriating to get called for nonsense, too. If you're waking me up at night, it had better be for something important. With many physician jobs, though, it is almost impossible to avoid call. If you choose any type of surgery, it is very likely that you will have to take some evening and weekend call. If you are in a very large group or program, you may have a "night float" system that covers evenings and/or weekends, but it is hard to totally avoid call. That being said, even as a surgeon, your call burden will be very different depending on your practice setting. If you want to make sure you are never on call, consider a specialty like emergency medicine where you take regular shifts rather than call. Many hospitalists do this, as well. (In case you are not aware, a hospitalist is generally trained in internal or family medicine and then hired by a physician group or a hospital to cover certain shifts in the hospital. I did not really learn about hospitalists until I finished residency.) ER physicians and hospitalists may work nights and weekends, but generally not in a call format. If call is something you see as important, talk to some of the physicians in specialties you are considering to see what their call is like as well as call options within the field. If you talk to a specialist at the tertiary care academic center where you are attending medical school, you will want to ask them what call is like for other people in that field since most physicians in the US do NOT work at tertiary care facilities.

Anatomical Factors: Eyes are tough for me. My eyes used to water when I watched my mom put her contacts in. In medical school, we had a week-long ophthalmology rotation in our core clerkships. On the first day, they put us in an auditorium with a movie theater-sized screen. We watched a video of a cataract surgery featuring a giant eye held open with a cage. When the colossal scalpel came for that eye, I knew ophthalmology was not for me. Yes, I probably could have trained myself to deal with it, but I was not interested. I have had to repair orbital fractures and perform an orbital exenteration with cancer surgery, so I can be professional, but they are not my favorite cases. If you are squeamish with something like that, you may want to avoid it. Additionally, the secretion issue I mentioned above is real. It takes certain types of people to deal with particular body parts/areas on a daily basis without being bothered. I smelled perforated bowel one day on my general surgery internship, and I never wanted to smell it again. But snot — no problem for me. You will definitely notice on your clinical rotations in medical school if you have an issue with something like this.

Patient Factors: Most patients are good people. I only end up meeting very few patients that I actually dislike (for a further discussion, see the section on Difficult Patients in my first book *Communication in Medicine*). However, there are certain groups of patients that some physicians do not want to see. My office space at a prior job was shared with a bariatric surgeon. Whenever we heard a medical assistant putting a screaming child in an exam room, he would turn to me and say, "I'm glad that one's not mine."

He was very happy that his practice did not involve pediatric patients. If you do not want to work with children (or their parents), do not choose a specialty where this will be part of your practice. Although quite different from children, "cosmetic patients" are another group that many practitioners dislike. There is no problem with dedicating your life to making someone look better. You might be able to make a lot of money doing it, and many plastic surgeons perform functional procedures in addition to their cosmetic cases. However, there is a common persona seen in many cosmetic patients. They are never quite satisfied with outcomes, always find something to complain about, and are very needy of their physicians. My plastic surgery colleagues in residency would often get paged repeatedly by cosmetic patients complaining that their nose was swollen after rhinoplasty or there was "a lot of blood" on the abdominoplasty dressing. When the residents would have these patients come to clinic to check on them, they would be healing just fine. If you are skilled at reassuring patients in these situations without pulling out your hair, you do not need to worry. We are all going to encounter high-maintenance patients, but there is a much higher percentage than usual among the cosmetic patients.

Flexibility: Some people feel like they need a lot of flexibility in their career, while others do not. If you need a lot of flexibility, you probably should not choose a purely surgical career. If you become a cardiac surgeon but decide 5 years into practice that you no longer like surgery, there is not much to fall back on. If you choose a medicine specialty, you may be able to go back and forth from clinic to hospital and full-time to part-time. Since ENT involves medical care and not just surgical procedures, some ENTs will choose to stop performing surgeries but still continue to see medical patients later in their careers. If you choose to become incredibly specialized, you may be limited by where and how you can practice. For example, if you choose to become an infectious disease physician focusing on tropical medicine, you may have a hard time finding a job in Alaska.

7. Notes on Individual Specialties

There are clearly too many medical specialties to have a discussion of the pros and cons of each in this text. However, in writing this book, I came across a book that I was able to download for free on just this topic (see Appendix 2). I have not read the book myself as it is definitely more information than I need at this point in my career, but I will briefly list for you some of the pros and cons of specialties – as I see them – as influenced by my training and interaction with colleagues. Unless otherwise noted, these specialties are each accessed through their own residency program right out of medical school. Some do have what's called a "transitional year" or an intern year which may not be directly related to the field, and may require a separate application (talk to a mentor in your field for more details). And yes, there are a lot of generalizations here. I think there are probably exceptions to almost everything I say in this section, but it is provided to give you some of the common perceptions of each major field.

Medicine group: This covers internal medicine (IM) itself and the specialties you can choose by first doing an internal medicine residency followed by a fellowship. IM graduates can become primary care providers or hospitalists. Numerous fellowships exist, including nephrology, rheumatology, gastroenterology, pulmonology, cardiology, genetics, geriatrics, allergy/immunology, hematology/oncology, endocrinology, infectious disease, sports medicine, and more. People in these fields generally like solving problems academically and working with patients. These may be brief encounters or life-long relationships. Pay varies widely across the specialties, as do interventional or "hands on" opportunities. Doing an IM residency allows you to get out in practice quickly (3 years), or to take extra time to specialize in one of many different fields.

Pediatrics: This is almost exactly the same as the internal medicine group, except you are dealing with children instead of adults. The residency, fellowships, and career pros and cons are pretty much the same. There are generally fewer pediatric specialists in a given field than the adult equivalents, but this is the main difference. If you like everything mentioned in medicine but you love kids, choose pediatrics. Pediatrics has a different "feel" to me than adult medicine. I myself and surgeons in general are sometimes frustrated by the way that many pediatric nurses, doctors, and child life specialists talk about their pediatric patients like they were their own children, and try to make the hospital a "happy place" rather than a medical facility. We never want to inflict unnecessary pain, but there is a reason the child is in the hospital and we need to prioritize the medical care of that child. If a child is sick enough that he has to be admitted to the hospital, he probably needs an IV (at least in my book). Although that's not "fun" for the child, it's likely to be medically necessary. Most medical students can quickly determine which demographic they prefer.

Family Medicine: If you like kids and adults, family medicine might be for you. Family medicine and emergency medicine are probably the two specialties where you get to do a little of everything. I would say family medicine leans more towards the "thinking" side, but many family medicine doctors do a lot of procedures, too. OB/GYN is incorporated into most (if not all) family medicine residency programs, so you even get to deliver babies. This is the best specialty for having longitudinal relationships, since you can care for a person from birth to death. You may become frustrated by "non-compliant" patients, but you generally have the best chance of any physician to change their behavior since you see them regularly. There is an element of triage since you will have to refer some of your patients to specialists, but you will be able to do a lot on your own. The pay is not as good as most other specialties, but you still make much more than most other professions. A lot of paperwork (disability, physical forms, etc) often falls to family medicine doctors and other PCPs (pediatricians, internal medicine doctors).

Surgery group: General surgery is the internal medicine equivalent of this group, in that you can practice general surgery right after the residency or pursue several fellowships. These fellowships include vascular surgery, thoracic surgery, colorectal surgery, endocrine surgery, minimally invasive surgery, oncologic surgery, and more. The surgery group also contains the surgical subspecialties of orthopedics, ENT, urology, neurosurgery, and plastic surgery.

Plastic surgery is unique in that it can be done as a residency straight out of medical school, or can be pursued as a fellowship after general surgery, ENT, or sometimes orthopedics. Oral surgery combines medical and dental school prior to the residency. Surgeons of all types generally have some call responsibilities that vary based on the specialty and practice. Most of us really enjoy being able to "fix" a problem by removing diseased tissue or repairing damaged or dysfunctional structures. The pay is often higher than many other medical fields. You may develop longitudinal patient relationships at times, but many surgical encounters are fairly short-lived. You need to have a high level of self-confidence to be a successful surgeon, as your patients need to trust you and you usually "lead the team" in the OR. You also have to be able to make quick decisions in the OR, and deal with complications.

OB/GYN: This is one of the most difficult specialties to avoid call, unless perhaps you subspecialize in something like gynecologic oncology. Malpractice premiums are generally quite high, as well. However, many OB/GYNs really enjoy their field. You get to work with young, generally healthy women at a very happy time in their lives. You can go the other direction, too, and do maternal-fetal medicine where you deal with the high-risk pregnancies. This is a unique field in that OB/GYNs spend a fair amount of time operating in the abdomen, but do not actually spend any time on general surgery services in their residency. Most surgical subspecialties have an intern year that incorporates at least some general surgery rotations. Even though ENTs and orthopedists will never operate in the belly, we are still required to spend time training in this area. Due to the absence of general surgery training, OB/GYN is considered by some to be a "semi" surgical field. OB/GYNs often perform a lot of surgeries, but it is a very different training pathway than general surgery.

Emergency Medicine: This is a great field if you enjoy working at a fast pace and you like multiple fields of medicine. When someone asks, "Is there a doctor on the plane?," they are really hoping for an emergency medicine physician. As a medical student, my top two choices for a career at the end of my core clerkships were ENT and emergency medicine. Emergency medicine is usually a great rotation for medical students because you get to do a lot — draw blood, suture lacerations, set broken bones, perform CPR, and generally use your diagnostic skills to treat potentially life-or-death situations. Even though it was a lot of fun, I realized it was not the career for me. I did not like the fact that some patients use the ED (emergency department) for primary care. I did not like the shift work at the time (although it may be better than call for some people). The adrenaline rush can be great when it's there, but it is hard to live like that all the time. One of my best friends from medical school chose emergency medicine. He works at at urgent care clinic now so gets to avoid both call and night shifts, but he misses some of the higher acuity cases he saw when working in a true ED. I am impressed by how much he knows about a lot of different topics, but ED doctors still have to rely on specialists in certain situations. Burnout is high in emergency medicine. Many of the physician administrators in hospitals and other organizations are former or "reduced-practice" ED docs.

Psychiatry: My first clinical rotation in medical school was inpatient psychiatry. I was so excited that I would finally get to see patients. Unfortunately, the psychiatrist I ended up working with was very jaded and didn't want the medical students to talk to patients. The students assigned to the other psychiatrist at the facility had a great experience though, since she was basically the opposite of my preceptor. If you enjoy learning about how the mind works and what happens when things go wrong, it seems to me that psychiatry could be a fascinating career. I really like to be able to reason with people and use logic (typical surgeon mentality), so inpatient psychiatry was not my field of choice. However, psychiatry gives you the chance to be creative in your solutions to problems, and you can build lasting relationships with patients. You have to be a good listener and have patience. Pay is generally moderate compared with other specialties, and the hours are usually pretty good.

Pathology: I didn't hear much about pathology in medical school, but I think it is an interesting field. There is generally limited patient contact, although some pathologists do their own biopsies. This is a great field if you really enjoy critical thinking and "hands-on" work, as you usually get to do both. Some pathologists have technicians who prepare samples for them, but many pathologists are called on to do their own processing, at least at certain times. As a surgeon, I enjoy getting to speak to the pathologist when I request a frozen section at surgery. It helps keep my skills sharp when I look at the tissue myself, and many pathologists I have met are great people. As a pathologist, you may be able to develop strong relationships with your surgeons and other clinicians, so you may not be off in a room with slides by yourself all day. On the other hand, if you like to be alone, it is generally easier to do this than in some other fields. Pathologists tend to have limited call, as well, and are paid fairly well.

Radiology: This field shares a lot with pathology in the way you interact with patients and other physicians. It also requires strong cognitive skills. Interventional radiologists spend a lot of time with patients, whereas diagnostic radiologists generally have very little patient contact. Radiology lends itself very well to telemedicine, which may give you more freedom with your career. On the other hand, it may be hard to leave work at work since you can (sort of) read a film from anywhere you have internet access. I did a neuroradiology rotation in medical school that was both fascinating and boring at the same time. I enjoyed learning from the radiologist, but it was sometimes hard to stay awake in a darkened room while watching someone else read films.

Dermatology: Dermatology is one of the most competitive residencies. I think this is because the pay and the hours are both quite good. Dermatology is generally conducted in an outpatient setting. Dermatologists can get additional training in Mohs surgery, but this is usually still done as an outpatient. Dermatology is one of the few fields where you get to see patients of all ages. Most medical schools teach you about dermatology in the histology course, but you do not learn much about it as a career. If you enjoy diagnosing and treating skin conditions, try to obtain dermatology experience early on since it is such a competitive field.

Ophthalmology: I already talked about my personal feelings about eyes, but I have nothing against ophthalmologists. They may even be in a close race with us otolaryngologists for the most difficult specialty name to spell correctly. There are a lot of specialization opportunities available within ophthalmology, and many of these are quite procedure-heavy. Ophthalmologists can have both longitudinal patients and brief patient encounters. The combination of good pay and great hours are hard to beat compared to other specialties. It's easier to do if eyeballs don't gross you out, though.

Anesthesiology: During my residency, the anesthesia residents seemed to be the happiest group of residents in the hospital. I don't know if a certain personality type is drawn to anesthesia or if it was just the character of that particular program, but I always enjoyed being around them. Most anesthesiologists spend their time in the OR, but there are other options available. For example, some will do pain medicine or critical care fellowships and spend their time in the outpatient clinic or ICUs. Anesthesia provides a nice combination of critical thinking and hands-on care. Anesthesiologists need to know how to react to emergencies, and physically apply their understanding of physiology and pharmacology. They intubate patients, place multiple lines/IVs, and perform nerve blocks. Call can be heavy, light, or none depending on the practice. Pay is quite good. The dynamics in the OR are strange in that the surgeon is referred to as "the captain of the ship" and the mantra is "blame anesthesia," even though surgeon and anesthesiologist are both highly trained professionals critical to the success of the operation. I have not seen any power struggles play out in the ORs where I have worked, but ENTs are often considered to have a better relationship with anesthesiologists than other surgeons since we "share the airway."

Neurology: This is its own residency, although it seems to share common themes with some of the medicine fellowships. I thought neurology was fun in medical school because it was kind of like detective work to figure out what was wrong or identify the "site of the lesion." However, I was frustrated because I felt like I could not really fix any of the problems. I could tell someone where they had had a stroke, but could not really improve their weakness.

Neurology is a hot area for drug development and research in general, so treatment options will hopefully improve.

8. Be Realistic

Now that you know a bit about most specialties, it's time for a reality check. If you barely passed your pre-clinical work and did not excel in the clerkships, it is going to be very hard to match in one of the very competitive specialties. You can improve your chances by doing research or excelling on away rotations, but don't put all of your eggs in one basket. Always have a backup plan. You don't want to have six figures of medical school debt and no way to pay it off if you can't match.

Chapter Three: Residency Selection

This is to help you choose your actual residency program once you have already chosen your specialty. Residency is where you will really learn the skills to practice in the field you choose. Residencies last from 3 to 8 years, depending on the specialty. Even within the same specialty, each residency program is unique. Your individual experience will even be different from your classmates due to your attitudes and interests. Whatever specialty you choose, you want to then select the residency program that personally prepares you best to practice that specialty.

1. Narrowing the List

If you are like me, you will not have your heart set on a particular program when you start. The only program you probably know much about is that at your medical school's home institution. You need to look at the websites of individual programs to at least learn the basics. Some specialties like ENT and plastic surgery have 100 or fewer residency programs, whereas others like family medicine and internal medicine have over 600. Since I was going into a "small" field, I looked at the list of all of the programs and asked myself geographically where I would prefer to live. I think this gave me a list of about 20 programs to start with.

If you do not have any geographic preferences or this does not narrow the list enough (e.g. you still have 200 programs left), you can try other factors. You may want to ask people you know in the field if they have any recommendations, either for programs they like or programs to avoid. It is best to know what you want in a program (see "What to Look For" below) before you ask them so they can give you the best possible advice. There is also a "Residency Navigator" tool from Doximity (see index for link) that allows you to compare residency programs. You do have to register with the site for full access, but it is free. A lot of their data was gained from surveys so there is limited objectivity. However, the recommendations you get from doctors at your institution are not going to be unbiased, either. Once you have a reasonable number of programs, you can look at each program's website for more details to help further narrow your search. If you cannot narrow it down before this step, you will just have a lot of websites to go through.

2. Broadening the List

If you have an initial list in mind that has too few programs, you will need to include more. Even if you have your heart set on one certain program, you need to have others as backup options. You can use the factors in the "narrowing" section in the opposite way to find more programs that interest you. If you only want to go to one of the top 10 residency programs in a given specialty, you may need to apply to the top 20 or 30 to match (but I have to say that exclusively using any type of published ranking is not an ideal way to choose a program).

3. Be Realistic

How many programs do you need to apply to? This is determined by two main factors — your specialty of choice and the strength of your application. You can look at statistics on individual program web pages and the Doximity site to get a sense of how you stack up against the average resident in a particular program. Your most helpful ally in this task is generally an advisor in that specialty. Ideally, it should be someone who is very familiar with the residency application process. At my medical school, all of the students interested in ENT met at least once with the ENT residency director to frankly discuss the application process. He told us how strong our application was, if we were likely to match in ENT, if we needed to bolster our application with additional research or other activities, the number of programs we should apply to, which programs were relatively "safe" or were a long shot for us, and the number of interviews we should try to get in order to have the best chance of matching in ENT. He also advised some of the students who had weaker applications to have a backup plan, such as taking a year off to do research or applying to a second-choice specialty for them, like general surgery. This meeting was incredibly helpful because the residency director provided honest information on a subject that most of us as medical students knew very little about. In a less competitive specialty, this might not be as important. I still think it is a great idea to try to have a meeting like this if you can. If there is not someone available in that specialty, you should at least be able to talk to your Dean's office to find a knowledgeable individual to help you in this arena.

4. What to Look For

Although you will be a pediatrician after completing any pediatrics residency, not all programs are created equal. I highly recommend making a list of factors that are important to you and determine how each program ranks according to each of your own personal criteria. You want to do some of this prior to applying to programs, and make sure you update it right after going on each interview. Once you have gone on multiple interviews, things begin to blur a bit and it can be hard to remember which detail goes with which program. This list will help you immensely in both choosing where to apply and determining your rank order list for the Match. Here are some of the factors I recommend and that I used myself.

Board certification: What percentage of graduates of the program pass their specialty board certification exam, and how many tries does it take them? In order to practice in most fields, physicians are required to pass their respective board exam after graduation. If everyone completes the residency program but is not able to pass the board exam, that program may not be worth your time. There may be extenuating circumstances, but this is pretty important since it may seriously limit your practice.

Fellowships after residency: How many program graduates do fellowships, and in which specialties? If you want to be a nephrologist but no one from a certain internal medicine program has matched in nephrology in the past 5 years, you need to be cautious. Is it just that no one has been interested in it, or are that program's graduates not competitive in the field? Conversely, if you want to practice "bread and butter" orthopedic surgery but every program graduate for the past 3 years has done a fellowship, that particular program may not support you in your goals.

Program completion rate: Do all of the residents who start the program complete the program, or what is the attrition rate? If a program is incredibly challenging or "malignant," residents may choose or be forced to leave without finishing. Residents may leave for other reasons, too, but you want to try to make sure that you can complete a residency if you start it.

Coverage of specialties: Most fields have multiple sub-fields, and you want to make sure all of these are covered within your residency. First, this is the best way to prepare you either for general practice in that field or to go on to the fellowship of your choice. Second, board examinations will be much easier if you have been exposed to all of the information they contain. For ENT, some of the programs I looked at were weak in facial plastics or otology. I ended up ranking those programs lower on my list than the ones that gave good exposure to each discipline within ENT.

Case load: This information can be harder to find than the above data, but you can still get it if you ask the right people. This is especially important for surgical or other procedure-based specialties, but you may also be able to find out in medical specialties how broad the patient exposure is at a program. Each surgical specialty has "key indicator cases" that cover a wide variety of procedures within the field. We discussed this data for each of our ENT residents in my residency program several times per year to make sure we had at least as many as the national averages. This data may be included in presentations at your residency interview. If not, you can always ask the residents about it. If they don't know how they are doing, it may be a sign that they are not getting enough cases.

Physical facilities: You do not need to have the most expensive state-of-the-art equipment or a shiny new building designed by a famous architect to get a good training, but you do need to make sure facilities are adequate. For example, it is quite helpful in an ENT residency to have a temporal bone lab where you can go to practice drilling for otologic surgeries. Not all programs have this, though. The ORs should have the equipment needed to perform all types of relevant cases. This may include a robot for certain specialties. You also want to have ICUs in order to learn to take care of the sickest patients. You should have access to a medical library, some sort of office space (usually a shared space for residents), and call rooms.

Training environment: Each residency program will have at least one hospital affiliation. This is often a tertiary care academic hospital, but some rural programs may have a community hospital instead. In many cases, it is beneficial to have multiple settings to get more diversity in patients and cases. My residency had the benefit of having an academic tertiary care hospital with an attached children's hospital, a community hospital, and a VA hospital. We did multiple rotations in each of these hospitals, and the patient population was quite different at each. I feel that this gave me a stronger training, but it is still possible to get a great training at only one hospital. Most specialists train at least in part at an academic institution. These hospitals usually have the most complex patients, and multiple consultants are often involved. It is good to be able to see these types of patients in residency, but emergency physicians and internists who are used to frequently calling consults may struggle if they get to a setting where these consults are not available. Some people may intentionally choose a "rural residency program" that emphasizes self-reliance and independence over calling consults. If you plan to practice in an underserved or rural area, this second type of program may be a better fit for you.

Resident morale: One of my medical friends posted on Facebook a cartoon that said, "The beatings will continue until morale improves." It was funny, but had a sad kernel of truth to it. Residency is a hard process. No one ever says, "I want to be a resident when I grow up." But it is important to look at the group of residents in the program and see how they react. Do they work together and support each other through the hard times, or are they out to get one another? Residents and faculty are going to be on their best behavior during interviews, so if they seem miserable even at that time, you should be wary.

Program fit: Do you like the people there? Could you see yourself working with them? I visited a couple programs that looked great on paper, but I could not wait to finish the interview so I could get out of there! I felt like I really enjoyed the people at two of the other programs I visited, and the rest were neutral. Since the two where I really enjoyed the people met all of the above criteria, I ranked them at the top of my list. You are going to be spending A LOT of time with your co-residents and faculty, so listen to your gut feelings about each place.

Diversity: This incorporates the traditional gender, racial, and cultural diversity, but you also want to look for training diversity. Did all of the faculty members train at the same institution, or do they come from a variety of places? In your training, you want to learn as many ways as possible to do a procedure or treat a disease. If all of your faculty trained at the same place, you will get less variety in this. You will still probably receive adequate training, but you want to be as well-rounded as possible. It is also nice to have a variety of ages in your faculty members, as training changes over time. You don't want all of your faculty to retire while you are there, either. In ENT, it is good to know about the history of the specialty and how to transilluminate a sinus when you don't already have a CT scan, but you also want to learn the newer technique of balloon sinuplasty.

ACGME accreditation: The ACGME (Accreditation Council for Graduate Medical Education) audits residency programs on a regular basis to try to make sure they are providing appropriate training. The ACGME gives each program a sort of "seal of approval" for a given length of time after it does a site visit. It also provides a list of deficiencies, some of which the program is required to correct within a certain time frame. Ideally, your program should be "fully accredited." This means that everything went well with the most recent site visit. If there are any issues, you should know what they are to make sure your training will not be compromised. If the institution does not volunteer this information, you can always check on the ACGME site (link in index).

5. What to Avoid

The biggest thing to avoid is going to a place that you despise. This may be because of the other residents, the faculty, the facilities, or the geographic location. If you already hate it going in, residency will not improve your opinion. Listen to your instincts. Even if the best program in the country loves you, don't rank them highly if you dislike the place.

Be wary of programs that seem unstable. This may be evidenced by faculty turnover, resident attrition rates, or accreditation issues. During my residency, the oral surgery program at one of our institutions was discontinued. They had lost faculty members to the point where they could not maintain their accreditation. This was a very difficult situation for the residents, as they had to try to find other programs to join partway through the training process. Programs usually do not end overnight. Make sure you are not seeing any red flags when you start your residency, as transferring is often quite challenging.

Chapter Four: Residency Application

Now that you know where you want to apply, how do you do it? The online application process through ERAS is fairly simple — fill out a bunch of forms, choose your programs, pay a lot of money, and write your personal statement. Residency programs will use some of the data you enter to narrow their list of candidates, so you want to have worked hard throughout school and on the application itself to make this data as positive as possible. This usually includes MCAT scores, medical school grades, and publications. If you don't look good here, the program may not even look at the rest of your application. If you do look good here, your application will be forwarded to a review committee. This is where you have a chance to make a difference with your personal statement.

1. The Personal Statement

The personal statement is important, but I think some people make too big a deal about it. The most important thing is to make sure it is grammatically correct. If you have typos or incomplete sentences, it projects an image that you don't care about your application. Make sure you have someone read over it to catch these types of issues. Make sure that the personal statement makes sense. You don't want to jump all over the place and lose your reader. You should use transitions between paragraphs and have a clear beginning, middle, and end. Also, you want it to be interesting in some way.

What should you include in your personal statement? After reading it, the program should have a sense of why you are pursuing that specialty. It doesn't necessarily need to be the focus of your essay, but you want it to be clear. You may want to include a short anecdote or story about a life experience or event within medicine that has pushed you toward that field, if relevant. Limited use of inoffensive humor is also effective. Don't simply list all of your publications or awards, as the program already has that from the rest of your application. If there was one research project or mission trip that you really enjoyed, you may choose to expound on that in the personal statement. Be smart with the stories or jokes you utilize. You don't want to come off weird, but you don't want to bore the reader to death. I don't know if it was true, but one of the faculty in my residency told me about a personal statement from a female applicant that started with a story of her helping her family castrate bulls on the farm. The faculty member was a little scared of this applicant, and it seems hard to see the relevance of this story to a career in otolaryngology.

Some programs require that you include why you are interested in that particular program in your personal statement. This may impair the "flow" of your statement, so get help from your writer friends if needed. If your personal statement ends with a summary of the reasons you are interested in your specialty, it is easy to transition to why you think a particular program will help you live up to the best of your ability within that specialty. If it ends with an amusing experience you've had, maybe you can relate something in that experience to the program (e.g. geography, interaction with others, subspecialty within field that is well represented in that program). If you are copying and pasting, be 100% sure that everything in this paragraph matches the program you send it to. If you apply to a Los Angeles program first and mention the great weather, make sure you change that section when you do your Michigan application! (I grew up in Michigan, so I know about the weather there.) I cannot tell you how many people hurt themselves by being careless in this area.

2. Applications and Interview Invitations

You need to be thoughtful in the number of programs you apply to. It is going to be very expensive and time consuming to apply to 50 or more programs (which I know some people do, especially for competitive specialties). The otolaryngology ERAS page now tells applicants that they must include a paragraph in the personal statement about why the applicant is interested in that particular program. This is partially to discourage students from sending out blanket applications. I talked to the program coordinator at my residency, and she was always frustrated by the vast quantities of applications that came in from students who clearly had no knowledge of the program. If you are not interested in a program, DO NOT APPLY TO IT. My advisor encouraged me to apply to

25-30 programs for the best chance of matching. I applied to the lower end of this number, simply because there were not 30 programs that interested me. I also managed to save a little money by submitting fewer applications. I have talked to some family medicine residents that only applied to 5-10 programs and had no problems matching, so the number really depends on your specialty and application strength.

Once you apply, there is generally a waiting period before interview offers start coming in. If you have not heard anything, check discussion boards to see which schools have already sent invites. For ENT, everyone used otomatch.com. For other specialties, you can do a Google search with "[specialty name] residency interview invites." People on these boards will list which programs have sent out invites and when. Users of these boards will also often post the interview dates for each program once they are known, so this can be helpful in planning your schedule. Some schools are slower than others in offering invitations. Also, even if you do not get invited in the first wave, you may still receive an invitation if an applicant invited in the initial group declines the offer. Do not contact a program over and over to check the status of your application. This will only annoy them.

There are some candidates who are so strong on paper that they will be offered interviews at almost all programs where they apply. You are also very likely to get an interview at your home institution and any program where you did an away rotation, as long as you did a good job. Other than that, it seems pretty random as far as which programs offer interviews to which candidates. The ENT residency director at my medical school told me that programs will sometimes choose candidates who have a geographic link to the area, as that candidate may have a stronger desire to be there. However, even though I grew up in the midwest, I got very few invitations to midwest programs. I was invited to all 3 of the programs in the San Francisco area, even though I had absolutely no California connection. The "strength" of the program did not always correlate with invitations, either. I got invited to some top tier residencies but not some of the schools I thought of as "safer" options. Many programs get so many applications from high quality students that it is really hard to choose who to interview. I recommend that you listen to your qualified advisor. You may not end up interviewing quite where you thought, but as long as you get enough interviews, you should match.

As the offers come in, you will want to limit yourself on the number of interviews you accept. Hopefully, if you have followed the advice of your mentor and this text, you have not applied to programs that do not interest you. When an interview offer comes in, then, you will want to accept it. It may happen that interview dates of two programs conflict with each other. If you cannot resolve the conflict, choose the program you prefer and make sure you let the other program know right away that you cannot attend so they can offer the interview spot to another deserving candidate. Also, if things change and you are no longer interested in a program, politely decline their offer as soon as possible. Most specialties are surprisingly small, and word gets around if you cancel multiple interviews or if you inconceivably no-show for an interview. You do not want this reputation at the beginning of your career.

If you happen to be invited for an interview at each program, you have somehow hit the jackpot. However, if your advisor said you only need to go on 10 interviews, do not waste your time and money going to 30 interviews. You will be exhausted, and will not perform as well as you could if you were more rested and focused. You are wasting that program's time if it is not near the top of your list. Also, you are taking an interview slot away from someone who may be more interested in that program than you. I ended up going on 9 interviews, and that felt like plenty by the end.

3. Residency Interviews

These are generally fairly informal, although many students stress about them. If you were offered an interview, it means that the program likes you. Their goal at the interview is to make sure there is not something wrong with you that does not show up on paper. Are you so incredibly shy that you won't talk to anyone? Do you have odd mannerisms or poor hygiene? As long as you seem fairly normal, you will probably be fine at the interview.

Even though the interviews are usually laid back, there are a few simple tips that are crucial to keep in mind. Be on time! Especially if you are going to an unfamiliar place, make sure you allow plenty of time to get there. You may need to check into traffic or construction issues. If you are delayed for some reason (e.g. your flight is cancelled), make sure you call the program to let them know what is happening. No-showing without explanation is probably the worst thing you can do. Dress professionally. Candidates usually wear business suits at residency interviews. Do not wear anything low-cut or overly revealing. Make sure you are well-groomed. Brush your hair, make sure you have showered, and clean your nails and hands. Do not wear strong perfume or cologne. Make-up and jewelry choices should be conservative. If you have a lot of piercings or tattoos, cover them if possible. This is not the best time to dye your hair blue. Patients are going to need to trust you as a physician, so you do not want to scare anyone away at this step in the process. Be polite at all times. If you are rude to the person at the front desk, the program director may hear about it. Use your manners with 'please,' 'thank you,' and holding doors. Smile and make eye contact when speaking with others. Do NOT incessantly use your smartphone. It looks much better to socialize with the residents, faculty, and other interviewees than to text all your friends at home. Plus, that is the whole reason you are there!

Your main goal at an interview should be to find out if the program is a good fit for you. You already should know a lot about the program structure and faculty from your pre-interview research. This involves thoroughly reviewing the program website, including learning about the faculty. It is especially helpful if you are given a list ahead of time of who will be interviewing you. At small programs, you often meet with a large percentage of the faculty, so you may have 8-12 interviews in the day. With larger programs, you usually only meet with 2-4 faculty and have fewer interviews. The interview is generally a half day to a full day. There is usually some sort of presentation on the information that the program wants you to know, followed by faculty interviews. You will also have formal interviews with residents at some programs. Most interviews have a social event before or after the interview. It is nice to attend this if possible, as you can interact with residents in a more relaxed setting. You do not need to wear your suit to the social event.

Some interviewers will just try to get to know you, while others will ask "tough questions." These generally deal with ethical issues, teamwork, and handling challenging situations. The interviewer may give you a scenario and ask how you would handle it, or make you give an example of a situation where you had to show patience, deal with failure, etc. It is helpful to read examples of some of these questions to prepare yourself. You can find lists online (see link in index) or in residency preparation books. The idea is not to prepare an answer you can recite verbatim, but to have ideas in mind so you do not waste all of the interview time trying to think up answers from scratch. If you are generally a nervous person, you may want to actually practice interviewing with a friend or mentor. Your medical school may also be able to help with this. Make sure you review everything you put in your application, as some of the interviewers' questions will likely come from information in your packet. I was asked multiple times about some of my research projects in various interviews.

In addition to preparing for questions you will be asked, you want to make sure you have intelligent questions to ask the interviewers. By the end of the interview process, I got tired of hearing, "Do you have any questions?" You want to appear intelligent and interested in the program, so don't just say 'no.' Good questions are those that you cannot find the answer to on your own. Most programs post their curriculum by year, so don't ask, "How much time do residents spend on cardiology?" You might instead ask, "I know that residents spend 2 months on cardiology in their PGY2 and PGY3 years. Is there an opportunity to get cardiology exposure prior to that?" This shows both that you have researched the program and that you are a go-getter. Another good question is, "I see that about 2/3 of your residents go on to do fellowships. Do they tend to get their top choices?" You can also ask about projected changes in the program, program goals, and strengths and weaknesses. There are going to be certain factual questions that you will only want to ask once (like fellowship matching), but the opinion questions can be asked of multiple people as each person might give you a different response ("What do you like best about this program?" "What do you wish you could change?"). Make sure you have some good opinion questions ready so you are prepared whenever you are asked if you have any questions. You don't always need to ask multiple questions, but make sure you show your interest.

Right after your interview, make sure you take notes so you can remember each program. As I mentioned earlier, it is helpful to have a chart so you can compare and contrast each program. You should also have a freehand section to mark down other details and impressions. Do this right away so you don't forget! You may want to go ahead and rank programs from top to bottom preference as you go along. Some people choose to send thank you notes after interviews. I did not do this, and I still matched. You may ask your program or colleagues what they think about it. Do make sure that you thank people for their time while you are there, as well as the chance to visit and learn about their program.

4. The Match

The Match is the allocation process for residencies in the US. After you apply and interview, you will need to make a rank list. Basically, you place in order the programs where you interviewed from top choice to bottom choice. If you absolutely do NOT want to train at a certain program, do not put it on your rank list. If you end up matching at any program on your list, you are basically obligated to go there or just not do a residency. (This probably violates some sort of labor law, but it is the way it is done.) You can use any of the factors mentioned above and include any others that you think of to make your list. I found that most of the programs where I interviewed had the nuts and bolts of a good training program in place, so I ended up ranking the two where I felt I really clicked with the people at the top. Your number one goal should be to get good training, but you want to be as "un-miserable" as possible while doing it.

Programs will also submit their rank list of all the candidates who they interviewed. I got to be part of this as a chief resident. It was an interesting process. All of the faculty involved in the interview process and the chief residents met after each interview session to rank the candidates. We then met at the end to combine all of the candidates into an overall list. There were some candidates who we all loved, and we put them at the top. We only had 3 spots per year, though, so even if we matched our top 3 candidates, there were still others we really liked. The difference between candidates #3 and 4 was minimal, but only 3 could be ranked to match. There were a few candidates who we generally disliked (usually from odd behavior at the interview), so we had to choose whether we would even rank them or not. The faculty and residents would discuss all of the candidates as they appeared on paper and in person.

Once the candidates and programs have each submitted their rank lists, a mysterious computer algorithm goes to work to determine "The Match." I was initially told that the computer gives the candidates' lists priority over the programs' lists. This would mean that if I chose Program A as #1 and Program A and Program B both put me as #1, I would go to Program A. I was later told, though, that the true goal of the algorithm is to fill as many residency positions as possible. This means that even if a candidate and a program rank each other highly, the candidate may end up at another program if doing so fills a spot that would otherwise be vacant. I do not know anyone that works for ERAS so I cannot verify this, but it seems true to me. It is potentially frustrating for the candidate and program if they do not end up together, but I don't know of a way to change the system.

Each spring, medical students anxiously await "Match Day." This is when the Match results are revealed to candidates across the country. Programs actually know if they have filled their spots a few days before this, but they are not allowed to tell candidates anything until Match Day. Most medical schools have a ceremony where they hand out the Match results to each student. This is a very emotional moment for most people, but remember that you will still be able to practice in your field even if you don't match at your top choice. If you don't match, you can participate in "the scramble" where you try to get into any open residency spot. A very small percentage of students have to scramble, but that process can be hectic. Make sure you know who in your medical school helps with that so you are prepared if needed.

Once you match, you can take some time to relax (finally). I recommend doing something you enjoy for at least part of the summer after you graduate, as it may be your last summer of freedom until you retire! Residencies technically start July 1, but you may have to do some orientation/training in the preceding weeks.

Chapter Five: Choices During Residency

This is a short chapter, because you do not get to make a lot of choices in residency about your day-to-day activities. ("What type of suture do you want to use to close the incision?" It will be whatever one the attending tells me to use. "Where do you want to go out for dinner tonight?" That's funny that you thought you'd be leaving the hospital before all the restaurants closed.) You will make important career decisions during this time as you look for your first job, but that is addressed in another section. In residency, you don't really have any say about contracts, salary, call schedule, or location. You do not have a lot of freedom in deciding how to spend your time. We will discuss the few things you ARE able to influence.

1. Your Attitude and Reactions

Residency will be hard. Some programs and specialties are more grueling than others, but I have not heard anyone say residency is easy. There are psychological and physical pressures. You are often sleep deprived and feel like you do not know as much as you should. There is frustration with the lack of respect you get from some patients and colleagues.

Although you cannot control these challenges, you can control the way you react to them. If you have a positive attitude, you will do a better job handling adversity. A few years ago, I read a book called *Learned Optimism* by Martin E.P. Seligman. While some of the "pessimism" he discussed sounded more to me like not taking responsibility for your shortcomings, I still appreciated the overall message of cultivating a positive attitude. If you struggle with negativity, you may want to read Dr. Seligman's book or one like it.

When I received criticism or negative feedback during residency, I found that the best way to respond was to avoid reacting. It was not helpful to be defensive. Later on, after the sting was gone, I would take time to think about what the person said. Was there some validity in the comment or were they just being mean? If the critique was legitimate, I would try to see how I could change my behavior to improve the situation. If the person was just venting, I tried to tell myself that.

2. Your Communication

The way you communicate with your patients, coworkers, and the outside world makes a huge difference in how you experience your residency (and life in general). I have definitely struggled with this at times, and residency was one of the hardest periods. Part of the challenge is facing new scenarios and new people while your role is constantly changing. Communication in medicine is such an important subject that I dedicated an entire book to it — entitled, conveniently enough, *Communication in Medicine*. I think every medical student and resident should read it to avoid some of my mistakes, but I especially recommend it if you have difficulties in this area.

3. Research

Many programs have research time built in. You generally get to choose your own research project. Sometimes you choose from a list of projects. In other cases, you may work with a faculty member to create your own project. Try to select something that interests you, as you will probably do a better job if you enjoy the work. Ideally, it is nice to get at least one publication out of your research. Make sure you discuss the timeline with your research mentor so you are likely to complete at least the majority of your work during the dedicated research block. You probably won't have a ton of spare time to wrap things up when you're back on service.

4. Electives

Some residencies have elective time (mine did not). Use this time to pursue an interest or further your career goals. If you are a pediatrics resident planning a fellowship in pediatric pulmonology, you might use your elective for a pediatric pulmonology, adult pulmonology, genetics, NICU, or ENT rotation to further your career. Or maybe you want to do a mission trip while you have the chance.

Try to talk to the residents who have gone before you to see which electives they found beneficial.

5. Tailoring Your Residency

While some residencies like mine literally have every rotation laid out for you, you still may have some options to tailor parts of the residency. In my residency, our only dedicated otology time was a four-month block in the PGY4 year. Since I really enjoyed it and had a talent for it, though, I worked with faculty to get more otology cases in my fifth year. At the community and VA hospitals, I made sure I was always in on the ear cases. I even had a few opportunities to do otologic procedures when I was on the head and neck service at the academic institution (e.g. when someone was out sick or on vacation, when we had joint otology/oncology cases, or when we just weren't as busy on the head and neck side). With these adjustments, I ended up as primary surgeon on many more otology cases than the national average. If you have a special interest or talent in a certain area, talk to your faculty and program director to see if you can cultivate it during the residency.

Chapter Six: Choosing Your Career

After completing residency, most people either do a fellowship or go into practice. There are also less traditional options you can pursue with the MD or DO degree. Some of the different career paths are discussed here. The first five can be done with or without a residency, and the rest require completion of a residency program. Feel free to be creative, too. I'm sure there are careers now that I've missed and there will be new ones in the future that can be done using your medical degree.

1. Research

You generally do not get as much research experience obtaining an MD or DO as opposed to a PhD, but you can still choose to work as a researcher after earning your degree. The benefits of becoming a full-time researcher include no call, not having to endure residency, and often a flexible schedule. Researchers generally do not make as much money as practicing physicians, and may have to compete for grants to fund their work. I would not recommend applying to medical school with the idea of becoming a researcher unless you want to do purely clinical research or do a joint MD/PhD program. However, if you are exposed to research during medical school and decide you want to devote your life to that, it is a perfectly reasonable option.

2. Teaching

Most physicians who teach do so in addition to their regular clinical practice, but you may be able to find full-time teaching opportunities after medical school. Like research, teaching does not pay as well as clinical work, but you have a lot more time off. Very few medical school instructors are full-time teachers, but depending on how much you want to work and how much income you need, this may be an option. I really enjoy teaching, but I think my teaching skills are best used in a clinical setting.

3. Administration

If you enjoy managing people, you should be able to find many administrative opportunities. These exist in hospitals, insurance companies, medical schools, and more. Some jobs will want you to have clinical experience before becoming an administrator or concurrent with your administration duties, but it is not always required. Many physicians have a negative impression of administrators since we as physicians do not like being told what to do in general, especially if it comes from someone who is not practicing in our specialty or practicing at all. However, administrators are not going away, so if you can effectively do the job, you may want to consider it. Some administrators have high incomes, while others are more modest.

4. Industry

Once you earn your medical degree, you may be eligible for advisory roles or consulting work with various companies. Many drug and medical device manufacturing companies like to have physicians who endorse and promote their products. The physicians may also help in product development or refinement. This is often done on the side by practicing physicians or as a second career after retiring from clinical practice, but you may be able to find opportunities right out of medical school.

5. Writing

Completing medical school gives you a marketable knowledge base. You may be able to write medical texts, articles, or blogs right out of school. General newspapers and magazines will often turn to a medical advisor before printing medical articles if they want to make sure they have the information correct. It may be hard to financially support yourself on this alone, but at least you don't have to take call. I have personally found that I really enjoy writing, too, so that is one of the main reasons why I have chosen to do some writing as a physician.

6. Fellowship

There are two main reasons to do a fellowship after residency. Some fields, like pediatric or medicine specialties, require a fellowship to practice in that area. The second situation is when you choose to do a fellowship to get more experience in a subspecialty. Most of the ENT fellowships fall into the latter category. You can legally do almost all ENT procedures straight out of residency, but you might want more experience within a certain area prior to trying to perform certain surgeries on your own.

A third reason that some people do a fellowship is to become more competitive in the job market. Fellowship training is required for some positions, and often encouraged for others. This is especially true of academic medicine, as many of the faculty members at academic hospitals have fellowship training. If you decide you want to pursue a career in academic medicine, you will probably do a fellowship if one is available. For some fields, this does not apply. If you are practicing something like general internal medicine or general pediatrics, you can still do this at an academic institution without a fellowship. Some programs will hire generalists in multiple departments, as well, to improve patient access and give their residents a broader training.

A bad reason to do a fellowship is because someone tells you to do it. One of my senior residents told me to do an otology fellowship. I did not want to give up the other aspects of ENT or spend additional time learning procedures I was not interested in. I could already do all of the procedures I wanted to do by the end of my residency due to the "tailoring" I discussed above. You need to determine for yourself if a fellowship is right for you, not just listen to someone else.

7. Academic Medicine

This is what most of us see during our residency, since a major component of academic medicine is teaching residents. This may be done at a community hospital rather than an academic medical center, but it still qualifies as academic medicine. Physicians who choose academic medicine usually do so because teaching is important to them. Most of the complex procedures are done at tertiary care centers, so physicians who want to do these procedures or focus on patients with rare diseases may be forced to work in academia. Physicians are usually employed (by a medical group, hospital, or university) and have a salary. There may be bonuses for production/RVUs, or the salary may be adjusted every so often based on the production. Academic physicians are usually busy as they have both patient care and teaching responsibilities. They may be required to mentor residents or medical students, give lectures, and participate in residency interviews. Research and/or publication may be required, as well. If you are in a large department, you will not be on call very often. It is also nice to have residents taking much of the primary call. The pay is usually lower in academic medicine compared to private practice. Most academic jobs are found in urban areas, since this is usually where large hospitals with teaching programs are located. Academic medicine tends to have more collaboration than many private practice settings, and many academic physicians enjoy this mental stimulation. You have easy access to CME lectures, and it may be easier to incorporate research into your practice.

8. Private Practice

Traditionally, private practice was the main alternative to academic medicine. Today, private practice takes several forms. In its purest sense, the physician owns his or her own business. The physician rents or buys office space, hires staff, deals with insurers, collects payments, and directs all aspects of her patients' care. Much of this is often handled by an office manager, but some physicians choose to do it themselves. This has become less common nowadays since it is tough to bargain with insurers on your own, financial stability is harder to come by, and most physicians have little expertise as businesspeople. The main benefit of having a private practice is the freedom you have to make decisions. If a certain staff member is not working out, you can fire him. If you decide you need another medical assistant, you hire one. If you need a new piece of equipment for the office, you buy it. When you do not own your practice, you have to get others to approve all of these undertakings, which can be difficult, time-consuming, or even impossible.

A second private practice option is to have a group practice (rather than the solo practice described above). This can be a single specialty or multi-specialty group (e.g. all gastroenterologists or gastroenterologists, pulmonologists, and rheumatologists). You still have decision-making power since you are a part owner of the practice, but the other owners have to agree with you. The bigger your group, the more likely you are to hire people to do some of the managerial or clerical work for you. These may include office managers, receptionists, coders, billers, nurses, surgery schedulers, and medical assistants. You are spending money on salary and benefits for these people, but it may allow you to increase revenue by spending more time yourself seeing patients.

Physicians in both types of private practice tend to earn more than academic medicine, but a lot of it depends on how you run your business. If you are shrewd, have a good patient base, and negotiate favorable contracts with insurers, you will likely turn a nice profit. If any of these factors are off, though, you may struggle financially. There is definitely more financial risk involved in private practice compared to other models, but the rewards of high levels of freedom and potentially high income may make it worth it for some. It is also harder to relocate geographically or to a different practice in the same area since you have a business to take care of.

9. Employed Position

This is becoming more and more common due to the challenges involved in running a private practice. In this model, a physician is hired by a hospital or a medical group. The physician usually has a guaranteed salary for the first 1-3 years of employment, then is paid based on production. Some employers continue this salary indefinitely without regard to production, but these are in the minority at this point. The employer takes care of hiring and paying staff, working with insurers, billing for services, and maintaining facilities. The main benefit is that the physician focuses on seeing patients without having to worry about the details of running the business. Also, if you decide you are not happy with your job or you want to relocate geographically for any number of reasons, it is much easier to quit than if you had your own practice. Employed positions generally pay better than traditional academic medicine, and can pay more or less than private practice.

The main downside of being an employed physician is that you have limited input in decision making. If you are upset with the performance of a medical assistant, you cannot just fire her. You have to tell your clinic manager about the problem, the manager has to see if he agrees, any unsatisfactory behavior has to be documented, remediation often has to be tried, and only then might the employee be terminated. You cannot set your own pay scale to try to attract higher quality employees. If you want any expensive equipment, you have to go through the capital approval process. Some things you want or feel you need do get done quickly, but this is not always the case.

Also, even though I said you do not have to pay attention to the business side of medicine when you are an employed physician, you probably should in some cases. In some of my prior positions, I was paid based on RVUs. If the insurer chose not to pay, it didn't affect my income. If I didn't code correctly, though, my income was definitely affected. I also kept track of my RVUs to make sure I was being paid correctly by my employer. Sometimes the coders would not use the codes I submitted, so I had to contact them at times to make sure they corrected things. As an employee, you are often required to go to certain meetings, too, so you are not 100% free from business matters.

10. Locum Tenens

This is another career path you may pursue after residency, although it was something I never heard about until after I finished my residency. This is basically "temp work" for physicians. You could also think of it as a "freelance physician." A hospital or practice may need a physician to fill in if one of their physicians leaves, gets sick, or goes on vacation, or if the practice is growing and they need more help. An assignment may last from a weekend to several months, and can be a single occurrence or a recurring opportunity. Some are "locums to permanent" positions, meaning that if you and the employer like each other, you might be able to take that job permanently. You are generally given a daily or hourly rate, and your travel, lodging, and malpractice insurance are covered. Physicians who know about locums will generally say that it pays well, but from my experience, it pays less per day than many full-time employed positions.

There are many benefits to locums work. You can choose how much you want to work. You may be able to make a full-time career out of it, or you may choose just to work a few months at a time or 1-2 weeks per month. You get the opportunity to see different places, and on someone else's dime. I would not want to pay for a condo in Waikiki, but it was a lot of fun to live there for a few months. Many people who do locums work feel appreciated when they go out on assignment. Although you are being paid, it is almost like you are doing a favor for the organization and the patients. As mentioned above, if you really like a place, there may be an opportunity to pursue a permanent position there. On the other hand, if you really hate a certain assignment, you are not tied into any long-term contract.

Locums work has its cons, too. Some people get burnt out by the traveling and constantly having to learn new systems. It is hard to build lasting relationships unless you have a recurring assignment. Locums physicians are sometimes considered to be lower quality than full-time doctors, but you do not have to let this apply to you if you want to do locums work. You can still maintain your patient care standards on your own. If you are not working very much, especially in surgical fields, you run a risk of having low case numbers that may make it harder to find employment down the road. Most facilities or locums agencies will help you obtain the license and credentials you need for each assignment, but it can be frustrating to fill out a lot of paperwork. The locums companies make a lot of money each time they fill a position, so I sometimes resented being their "cash cow." Also, locums work is not guaranteed. You may have a hard time finding assignments that you want. This type of work is challenging if you really like to plan ahead, since most assignments are only confirmed 1-3 months ahead of the start date.

If you are interested in locums work, do a google search for "[your specialty] locums." This will pull up websites where you can search for work yourself, as well as locums companies that do the work for you. Some people choose to do locums right out of residency, but it is also a way to keep involved in the field after leaving a full-time position. Some physicians will do locums work as a transition toward retirement. I have done several different assignments over the past few years. It was great to get to live and work in Hawaii and Alaska, but I also experienced a number of the frustrations mentioned above. I wrote a blog about it on a friend's website (see index), and you can find a lot of other articles online, too.

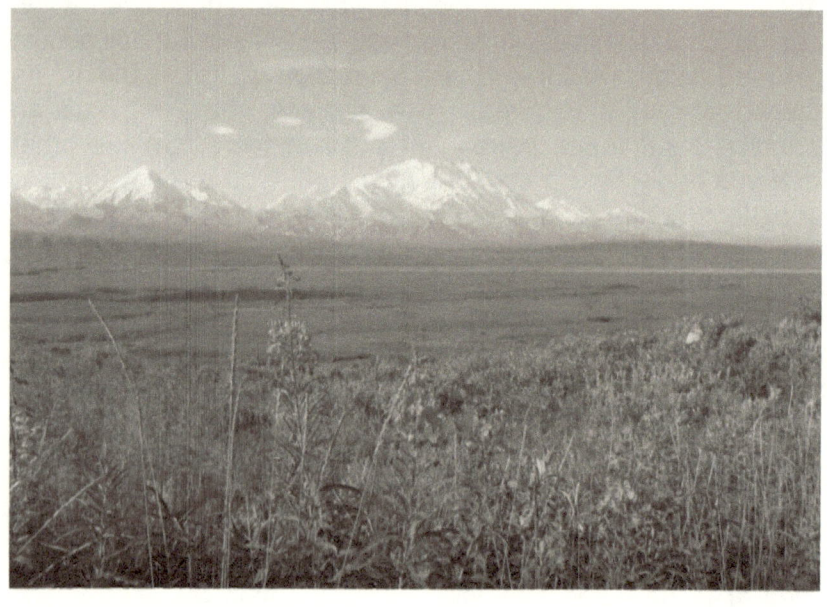

Denali with fireweed flowers – one of my days off working locums in Alaska

SECTION TWO: Getting the Job

In a sense, this is what you've been working toward your whole life. College, medical school, and residency have all been preparation for getting a "real" job. Yes, you get paid during residency, but the pathetic $12/hour I calculated for myself in intern year in the face of medical school debt, painful hours, and a high level of responsibility was not too encouraging. Unless you've done a non-traditional career path, your first job out of residency will be where you really need to know about contracts and employment options. Good physicians can be hard to come by in certain specialties and geographic locations, so you will hopefully find yourself in a position where the employers are really looking for you and not the other way around. You want to make sure you get the job you want, though, so this section will try to help you do that.

This is mostly aimed at physicians choosing to work as employed physicians rather than starting their own solo practices. The majority of physicians currently either work as part of a group practice or are employed by a hospital or medical group. I have never started my own practice, so I cannot speak as an expert on that. If you are interested in starting your own practice, I would highly recommend speaking to other people who have done it and reading up on business practices. I will definitely address business aspects of medicine later in this book, but it will not be enough to run your own practice. Some of the information in this section (e.g. licensing, credentialing) is useful for all physicians, regardless of practice type.

Chapter One: Preparing Your Application

Many people think that all you need to get a job is a decent CV. You definitely need one, but you will help yourself immensely by taking some other steps, as well.

1. Check your "internet resume"

When you do a Google search with your name (or its variants), what do you find? Is it a story about your mission trip to Africa, or the police blotter with your most recent misdemeanor? It is clearly better to avoid committing crimes in the first place, but you want to know what is out there so you are not surprised when you are asked about it. Lying is always a bad idea, but make sure you have an explanation for your past behavior.

While you generally cannot change public records after the fact (do not add hacking to your criminal list!), there are negative things on the internet that you can change. Clean up your Facebook and other social media accounts to remove any negative pictures (drinking, nudity, etc). Check your comments and posts to make sure any derogatory, racial, or just plain mean opinions are not out there for your employer to view. Many employers report that they do these sort of Google searches and check social media on their applicants.

You may also want to consider creating a strong Linked In profile. This seems to be more popular in business careers than medicine, but if the employer looks, you will be received favorably if you have taken the time and effort to create a good page. Most applications do not include photos, so Linked In is also a place where you can post a smiling, professional photo of yourself for the employer to see. If you just fill out the basic details, though, this strategy can backfire. You don't want to look like you are too lazy to complete a project, even a small one like a Linked In profile. You can also highlight factors or provide links that would not fit in the format of a CV. For example, in the Projects section of my Linked In profile, I was able to write a description of my book and include a link to its website.

2. The Curriculum Vitae (CV)

I watch a cooking show at times, and they have mentioned "haricot vert" on multiple occasions. Eventually, one of the show's participants admitted that it was a fancy term for green beans. Haricot vert and green beans may not be exactly the same, but for most of us, the differences are insignificant. The same is true with the CV versus the resume. Traditionally, the CV is for academic careers, while the resume is more for businesspeople. I think the biggest difference is in the research/publication section. A resume usually has a page limit, whereas a CV will get longer and longer based on how much you have published. Also, a resume is sometimes more "skills-oriented" whereas a CV is more "data-oriented." This means that you generally do not list your skills on a CV, but you may be able to comment on them under some of your accomplishments.

A CV needs to have your contact information (name, address, e-mail, phone number), education/training, medical work history, and publications. Putting the first four items in this order is fairly traditional. After addressing these factors, you may also choose to include other information. This includes research activities, volunteer projects, awards/honors, teaching activities, society memberships, presentations, or academic courses. Tailor this portion based on your own personal history and the job to which you are applying. For example, if you don't have any volunteer experience, don't make that a section on your CV. If you are applying to a position where you plan to do significant research, make sure you list your various research activities even if they have not resulted in publications. Many examples of professional CVs. are available online for free, so feel free to browse the web for additional ideas.

Make sure you proofread your CV. Spellcheck will help, but it cannot catch commonly misused homonyms ("their/there/they're" and "your/you're"). It helps to read it out loud to yourself, and also give it to someone else to read. If you cannot even use proper grammar, punctuation, and spelling on your CV, a potential employer will not be impressed.

3. Cover Letter

Some jobs will ask for a cover letter, and some will not. Either way, it is helpful for an employer to know why you are interested in that particular company. The main goals of a cover letter are to show why you want that job and why you would be good for that job. For example, when I applied for a job in northern California, my cover letter included the information that my husband was applying for a university position in the adjacent town and that I had enjoyed visits to the area to see the Redwoods and the coast. I also spoke about my experience with a broad variety of ENT problems in an area with limited resources, since this was the type of ENT doctor the practice was seeking. If you have family ties to an area, you want to be sure to mention that in a cover letter. An employer wants you to stick around after they hire you, so it is definitely a plus to the employer if this is the case. If a position has certain needs beyond just the type of physician (e.g. ENT, emergency medicine physician, pulmonologist), try to explain why you are a good fit. If you have experience in restructuring your residency curriculum and the employer is trying to start a family medicine residency, telling them about your work makes you a more desirable applicant. If you are a general surgeon who had a very strong oncology training in residency, you may want to highlight that fact.

The cover letter is your opportunity to connect with the person (or people) reviewing your application on a more personal level. Do not just list publications or research from your CV. Focus on the topics discussed above – why you want them and why they should want you. If there is anything 'unusual' in your background (malpractice suits, gaps in practice, etc.), you may or may not want to mention it in your cover letter. You don't want to try to hide anything, but you don't want to scare an employer away. For example, I took 5 months off between two of my jobs at one point. During this time, I was working on contract negotiations and the licensing/credentialing process for my new job, waiting to hear on a job for my husband, taking time to think about what I really wanted out of my career, and pursuing non-medical interests (which included hiking to the bottom of the Grand Canyon – which I highly recommend to anyone who loves the outdoors and has the stamina to do it!). Medical applications usually ask you to explain any practice gaps of longer than 3 months. I just stated, "I took 5 months off between practices to get ready for the new practice and pursue non-medical interests." No one expressed any concerns to me about that.

You can talk more about what you want in a position in the cover letter, too. I recently decided that I want to work part-time in a location within driving distance from my home, as my husband is tied to a job in a city where there are no good employment opportunities for me. All of the positions I found advertised were for full-time employment. I decided to go ahead and apply to some of the positions, but I told them in the cover letter that I wanted to work part-time there (1-2 weeks per month). Some of them replied back that they were only interested in full-time, but others have chosen to work with me.

As far as structure, the cover letter should be written in complete sentences, usually in a conversational (but professional) style. It should be no longer than 1 page. Ideally, you should try to address the cover letter to the person who will be reading it. This is often the partners (or senior partners) in a practice, a chief administrator in a hospital, or a physician recruiter. Again, make sure you check for proper spelling and grammar after writing the letter. If you are modifying it for different jobs, make sure it fits each job. If you still have questions, you can search for sample cover letters online.

4. FCVS

FCVS stands for Federation Credentials Verification Service, and is run through the Federation of State Medical Boards (FSMB). Basically, it is a repository of your official educational documents that you will need to provide to each state in which you apply for a medical license. Some states require that you use FCVS to submit your information, while others allow it as an option. There is a fee of several hundred dollars to establish your initial file, and additional fees each time you need to update information and send it out to new states. The initial process usually takes several months, and an "update" often takes 1-2 months. You might get lucky and things will move faster, but it is helpful to start this process as early as possible, especially if you know you will be practicing in a state that requires FCVS (see website in index). If you are practicing in a state where FCVS is optional, you can determine the cost in obtaining the documents yourself vs. using FCVS. This will usually include USMLE scores, the official medical school transcript, and verification of post-graduate training. The nice thing about FCVS is that it claims to store your information permanently, so you do not have to get the same official documents over and over. However, if you are not required to use it, it may be less expensive to do the legwork yourself. Some positions will reimburse you for fees associated with FCVS or obtaining documents, so you may want to check with your potential employer.

5. State Medical License

Each state you practice in will require you to have a medical license for that state. Applying for a state license is very annoying, as it is time-consuming, repetitive, inefficient, and expensive. (At least that has been my experience.) It can take anywhere from a few weeks to a few months depending on the state and the license type. If you are working with a locums company, they will often do a lot of this work for you, so that can be helpful. If you are working in an underserved area (see link in index), you may be able to pay a lower fee for the license and/or have it pushed through the system faster. The application for your medical license may occur before or after you actually apply for specific jobs, but you don't want to be delayed in starting a job because you have not yet obtained your license. If you know for sure what state you will be practicing in, you can start the state license application early in the process. Do a Google search for "[your state] medical board" and you will find the link to your individual state's requirements. You can have multiple active state licenses at the same time (e.g. if you live near a state boundary and have offices in more than one state, or if you work in multiple states with part-time or locums work). You just have to fill out repetitive paperwork and pay more fees. If you happen to work at US government facilities (i.e. VA hospitals or Indian Health Service (IHS)), you can generally use a license from any state.

6. Pharmaceutical License

Once you have your state license, you will then need to apply for the pharmaceutical license(s). This always starts with the DEA license (Drug Enforcement Administration). You will have had a training DEA license for residency, but will need your own personal DEA once you are actually out in practice. Guess what – this involves filling out more forms and paying more fees! In addition to the federal DEA, some states require a state pharmaceutical license to be able to prescribe medications in that state. In my own personal experience, it is sometimes difficult to determine if a state has that particular requirement. I obtained a medical license first in New Mexico, which did have its own state pharmaceutical license. Then when I applied for a license in California, people did not know what I was talking about since California only requires the DEA. You should be able to check with the medical board of your state and/or the people you will be working with at your job to determine what you need.

7. Review of Application Preparation

When I applied for my first job, it took about 9 months from the time I was offered a job to the time I was fully licensed. I had no idea it would take this long. Also, the administrative assistant assigned to "help" me in this process was not actually helpful. Since she worked with physicians all the time, it seemed like she would know I had to have the state license before I could do hospital credentialing (the process where the hospital where you will work reviews your documents to grant you privileges and have you approved by their insurers). However, she stressed to me how important it was to fill out my hospital credentialing packet (which was at least 50 pages long) ASAP to get it turned in, only to find out after I had done so that they couldn't do anything with it until they had my state license information ... which I hadn't filled out yet since I was working on the credentialing packet. Subsequent jobs have been faster, but have still taken at least a few months. The above steps provide an outline to show you what you need to do – and in what order – to be able to work after residency. The actual interview for your job will happen somewhere between CV preparation and hospital credentialing. It depends on your specific timeline, state, and employer.

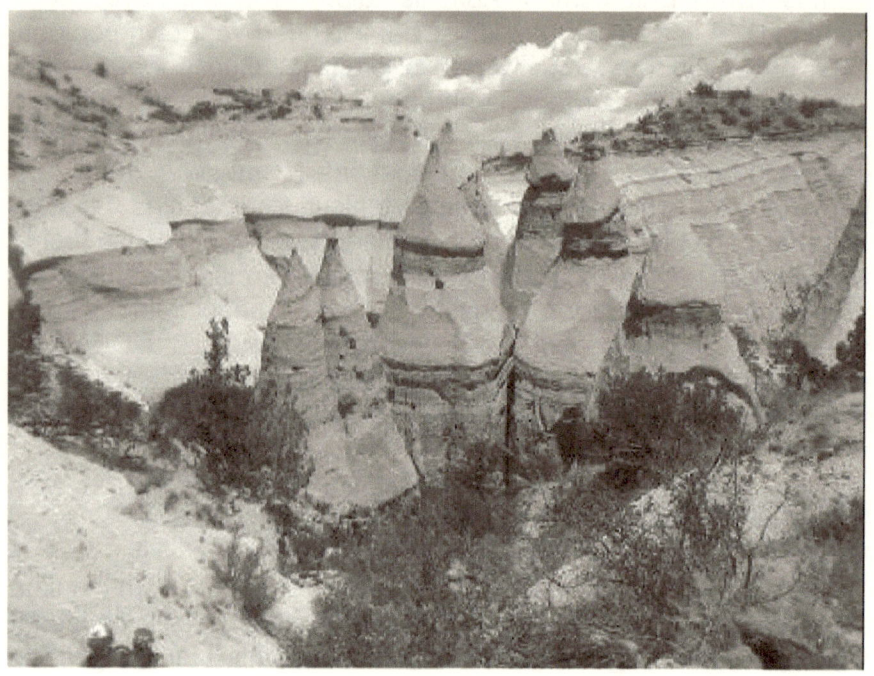

New Mexico – a stunningly beautiful state, but also "the land of mañana"

Chapter Two: Applying for Jobs

Now that you are prepared to apply for a job, you need to actually find a job to apply to. Sometimes jobs will just fall into your lap, but you usually have to put some effort into the search yourself.

1. Ways to Find a Job

There are multiple useful resources you can use to find a job as a physician. I will briefly discuss them, moving from easier methods to more challenging methods.

Work where you completed or are completing your residency: You already know the people and the environment. Being an attending physician in a practice vs. a resident physician is different, but you know more about this job than you would any other job to which you apply. If your department is looking to hire someone with your qualifications and you think you would like to stay, it can be a win-win situation. You will still do a formal interview and should ask the same questions you would ask at another place, but this is definitely one of the easiest job search methods.

Apply for advertised jobs: When I was a resident, I somehow started getting e-mails advertising ENT jobs at my work e-mail address. The e-mails came from several different companies, but I don't remember the names of the companies or how the e-mails started. If you get e-mails like this in residency, it may be useful to go through them. This is actually how I found my first job out of residency. I used other methods, as well, but my experience shows that this can work. In addition to unsolicited e-mails, jobs are advertised in medical journals (e.g. *NEJM* and specialty-specific journals). Print journals may not be completely up to date since there is a time delay with submission and printing, but you might still find good leads in the journals. Many journals have updated online job listings, too, so you may want to look there. There are various job search sites you can use (see index) to view posted jobs. Some allow you to search without entering any personal information, whereas others make you fill out a profile. Filling out a profile is not necessarily bad, as you can generally set your e-mail preferences to inform you of new jobs that fit your interests vs. limiting the number of e-mails you receive. I would NOT recommend supplying your personal phone number unless you know how it is going to be used and are okay with that. In addition to nationwide sites, simply doing a Google search for "[desired location] [your specialty] job" can reveal helpful leads.

Use a recruiter: There are both internal and external recruiters. Internal recruiters work for a particular hospital/health system and should know a lot about the potential employer. You usually will not have access to them unless you are applying to a particular job, as they will often be the contact people on job postings. Conversely, when most people think of recruiters, they think of external recruiters. These people work on their own or for a hiring company and help connect you with opportunities at a variety of places. They are sometimes unflatteringly called "headhunters," and their help can be both good and bad. I would recommend limiting an external recruiter's access to you (i.e. consider separate e-mail address or phone number), or at least make it very clear when they should be contacting you. Some recruiters abuse the privilege of having your information and contact you frequently about jobs in which you have no interest. However, they may know about opportunities you would not find on your own. External recruiters are generally paid a commission by the hiring company when they find a candidate but may not know much about the organization or location since they can be based anywhere. Locum tenens companies can almost be considered a type of external recruiter since they are hired by businesses to find candidates.

Pick a location and search for practices: This is actually what I did when looking for my first job out of residency. It involves more work on your part, but I think it provides a more exhaustive search and can lead to a more personal connection. This works best if there are only a few (or even 1 or 2) cities you are looking at, or if you are looking at smaller cities. Albuquerque was a place I was very interested in, so I did a Google search for "Albuquerque otolaryngology" and its variants (ENT, otolaryngologist, ear/nose/throat) and found the dozen or so ENT physicians in town. I determined the 4 different practices they worked at based on the business addresses (as well as a couple solo practices), and contacted all of the group practices to see if they were interested in adding a physician. Before doing this, I did a little internet research into each group and had my CV and cover letter prepared. Only one of the practices was actively advertising for an ENT, but all three others said they were interested and I ended up interviewing with all four. A lot of practices feel or know that they are understaffed, but may not have posted formal openings in places where you can find them as a job seeker. This strategy may not be feasible in a city that already has 80 pediatric practices (or 954, which is what my Google search tells me about New York City!), but it might still be helpful to check to get a sense of your options – or competition.

If you use this method, you will essentially be "cold-calling" the practices. Practice what you are going to say on the phone. I always listened for the name of the person answering the phone in their greeting. I would then say something like, "Hi [person's name]. My name is Kim Kinder and I am an ENT doctor interested in working in [city name]. May I please speak to your practice/office manager?" Be prepared for a variety of responses. The receptionist may directly connect you, give you another phone number, ask you to call back, or tell you they are not hiring. Once I got the right person on the phone (whether it was a practice manager or an internal recruiter), I would again introduce myself and ask if they were looking to add a physician to their practice. I was prepared to say why I was interested in the area and their practice, and what skills I could bring to the table. Most asked me to send a CV if they were interested. If they told me flat-out that they were not interested, I still asked if I could send a CV in case something came up in the future. I don't think I had anyone say no to that request. I've actually had some of these people contact me down the road when a position opened later on. If you are applying to a physician-owned practice, you may be talking to a physician for this rather than an administrator. Be polite to everyone, and make sure you know whom you are speaking with.

Networking: You may think your specialty network is pretty small when you start looking for jobs, but it is amazing to me how many connections I have found over the past few years. I did not utilize professional networking on my first job, but it has helped on late endeavors. I found an opening for a locums position in Hawaii, and remembered that one of my co-residents had found a job in Hawaii. I contacted him, and I think he put in a good word for me, which helped me in obtaining the desirable position. If you are flexible on where you land, you can ask your attendings or colleagues if they know anyone looking for jobs. Having a recommendation from a trusted individual can help you land the job, and if the person likes you (which we hope is the case!), they are unlikely to recommend a job where they think you would not be happy. You can look up where virtually anyone trained or went to school, so ask for insight and/or a peer reference if you are applying at a hospital or city where someone you work with has been.

2. The Actual "Application"

This varies from job to job. If you find an actual online posting, there is usually a form to fill out and/or a person to whom you send your CV. Make sure you READ THE DIRECTIONS and do what they ask. These things are usually not complicated, but it looks pretty bad if you can't follow simple instructions.

During the application process, there is often some back and forth. Make sure you are prompt in replying to any communications. You do not need to cancel your week-long camping vacation, but make sure everyone knows you are out of town so they do not give up on you when you don't answer immediately. Have an "out-of-office" reply on your e-mail or change your voicemail message to let people know how long you're going to be out if it's longer than 1-2 days. Be polite to everyone you speak with, as well. If you are a jerk to the receptionist over the phone, he might complain to his co-workers, and you may be less likely to get the job. Or even if you get the job, the staff members may remember the way you treated them and not work as hard to help you out. Use good e-mail etiquette, with proper salutations. Start the message with "Dear Dr. Lopez" or "Hi, Mary" rather than jumping right into the subject. Thank people for what they have done or what they are going to do for you.

A potential employer will usually ask for references at some point during the process if they are interested in you. Choose people who know you well and are likely to say positive things about you. Always ask the permission from a reference before you list them. It is also helpful to tell your references about any positions you are applying to and that you expect they might be contacted. Some job hunting books encourage you to seek recommendation letters from your references. I have not found this helpful, as it seems like each employer has a different way to contact the references. Some do a phone interview, some e-mail a form to fill out, and others ask for an actual letter. Unless you know that your potential employer wants a letter, I would not ask a reference to write one, as you may be asking them to do extra work. Always thank your references for volunteering to be your reference. (And on the flip side, try to say yes to your colleagues when they ask you to be a reference for them, as long as you have genuinely positive things to say.)

Chapter Three: The Job Interview

The next step is usually an interview. Some places may start with a virtual interview, or you may go right to an in-person interview. We talked a lot about interviewing in the residency interview section, and job interviews are similar. The company wants to make sure you are a presentable, sane, personable human and that you would be a good fit for each other. If there are other people applying for the same job, you may have to sell yourself more, but don't try to be someone you are not. That will not make anyone happy.

My experience was that the potential employers paid for my travel, lodging, and transportation for interviews. Sometimes they would book travel themselves, and other times would reimburse me. The person arranging the interview for you will usually volunteer this information, but if they do not, you can ask, "Does [name of organization] arrange travel, or do I do that myself?" I do not know if physician job hunters sometimes have to pay for travel themselves, but you might want to ask colleagues in your specialty about that if a company is not offering to pay for it. This type of thing can vary among specialties and geographic regions.

For both video and in-person interviews, make sure you are prepared. BE ON TIME. Allow extra time for the unexpected weblink problem or traffic jam. If you know you are going to be late, make sure you call and let the people know. You should be properly groomed and attired. Smile and make eye contact. Listen attentively and be polite. Silence your phone and only get it out in the privacy of the restroom. The organization wants you to be focused on them during the interview period.

You will usually be given a tour of the hospital and/or clinic. If you need certain equipment to do your job, the tour is often the best time to find out what is already there. As an ENT, I want to know what types of microscopes they have in the OR and clinic, as well as the availability of sinus CT navigation equipment and lasers in the operating room. Don't assume that a potential employer will have everything you were used to from residency. If you find that certain large capital items that you would need to do your job are missing, ask if they have plans to purchase the equipment (and then follow up in your contract – see next chapter). If you are mainly working in inpatient services, see what your office space, call room, and patient rooms are like. Is this a place you could work every day, or are you stuck in a dark hole? In your clinic, you will learn how many exam rooms there are, and how many exam rooms you will have for your patients. In busy practices, it is ideal to have at least 2 exam rooms per physician so you can be seeing one patient while the next one is being prepped for you. Many practices have space limitations, and you want to know what you are getting into.

In addition to seeing physical spaces, you will likely meet multiple individuals. I break these into two groups – people you will work with on a daily basis, and administrators. For practices with an outpatient component, your office staff will include receptionists, medical assistants, nurses, office managers, and additional clerical personnel (e.g. surgery schedulers). You may also have other physicians or mid-levels in your office. You generally don't get much time to speak with all of these people on your interview, but try to get a sense of general attitudes or any discord. Some offices will do an interview luncheon where the whole office is invited. This is a great opportunity for you to see how people actually get along with each other. I can say from experience that it is not fun to be in an office where no one likes anyone else. A good question to ask is how long various people have worked there. If there is a lot of turnover, that may be a red flag that something is wrong with the office.

If you will be working with other physicians or mid-levels on a daily basis, try to meet as many of them as you can. Being on the other side of this, when someone comes to interview where I work, I always like to meet with them. First, I want to know what they would be like as a colleague. Second, I want them to have as much information as possible to make the right decision. It is not helpful for anyone if they accept the job and quit a few months later so you have to start with a job search all over again. Companies usually try to schedule interviews when the doctors are going to be around. Ask what they like about working there and what some of their frustrations are, or things they would like to change. I would hope that most physicians are going to be honest with you, but I have unfortunately met a few who are less than transparent. Physicians are usually your most helpful source of information as to what it's going to be like to actually work there, since they're doing the same job you're going to do. If a physician has recently left the group or their absence is not explained on interview day, casually ask about the person if it seems appropriate. It could be totally innocent, or could be another red flag.

The office/clinic/practice manager is another important person to meet. You will usually have some one-on-one time with him or her. This person manages the office staff and is generally your "go-to" person for problems in the clinic. If you are being hired for an inpatient position, there should be some hospital equivalent of this person for you. A good clinic manager is incredibly helpful in making your job run smoothly. One of the reasons I chose my first job was because I was impressed with the clinic manager. (She unfortunately moved back to her home state within a year of me starting there, so that was a big disappointment!) You'll want to ask what things have changed recently in the office (e.g. improvements that have been made) and plans for any future changes. This may bring up both pros and cons that might influence your decision.

You might meet with hospital bigwigs, like the CEO or CMO. The questions about recent changes and upcoming plans are useful again here. If you have any serious concerns about hospital structure or other issues, you may consider bringing them up, but you do not want to come across as a negative person. However, if (for example) you learned that between the time you applied to a position and went to your interview that the hospital lost its accreditation or was bought by a new company, these are legitimate discussion topics. You may also have a meeting with someone to go over benefits and/or a contract. I recommend listening to them and making sure you get contact information so you can ask questions that might come up later. Benefits and the contract are important in making your decision, but not as crucial on your interview day.

There is often some sort of social event, like a dinner with other physicians. This is a great way to get more insight into the practice outside of the work environment. Significant others are sometimes invited, so ask about this if you are traveling with someone. Alcohol is often available, but do not drink to excess. Do not order the most expensive thing on the menu, unless everyone else is. This is still part of your interview, so don't do or say anything you wouldn't want a hiring committee to hear.

Especially if you are going on multiple interviews, take notes close to the time of your interview. You should include things you liked, things you need to follow up on if they weren't clear, potential areas of concern, and overall opinions. This will be helpful information when you are making decisions later on.

You might be given an actual job offer during the interview. Do not worry if this does not happen. Each company handles things differently. If you weren't given a job offer during the interview, ask when you should expect to hear from the organization and/or who to contact for the next step. If you are given the job offer, it is not advisable to accept right away. It is expected that you are going to need some time to review the contract.

Chapter Four: Contracts

My residency "contract" was a laughable document. It was a single 2-sided sheet of paper that basically said that the hospital would pay me a sadly low amount of money if I did what I was supposed to for the next year. I had to sign and date on the back page, and that was it. The physician employment contract is a very different document. My first one was about 25 pages, and my lawyer was impressed that it was "succinct." The next one was over 50 pages long. I don't know how they actually manage to write that much – a lot is made lengthy by "legalese" – but it sure seems like it becomes more complicated than it needs to be. That being said, you need to be prepared for what should be covered in a contract and what the important terms mean. I think most people hire a lawyer to review their employment contracts (or at least the first one). I did that, and I think it is a good idea for everyone. You might have to pay several hundred to a thousand dollars, but it is usually worth it. Knowing about contracts ahead of time will likely save you some money on legal fees since lawyers usually charge by the hour, and you won't need to ask quite as many questions. This chapter will first cover the different parts of the contract, and then talk about contract negotiation. As a reminder, this book is NOT a substitute for hiring a lawyer.

1. Offer letter

Before getting the actual contract, you will often receive a 1-2 page document. This might be called an offer letter, job offer, face sheet, or fact sheet. It is basically a "letter of intent" that lists some of the main points of the employment agreement. This may include salary, length of employment, conditions of employment (i.e. completion of background check, licensing, and credentialing), call frequency, practice location(s), productivity bonus information, a list of benefits, time off per year, or other details. You sometimes have to sign this to get the actual contract. This does NOT legally bind you to work for the company. However, the idea is that by signing this sheet, you are agreeing to work with them if you come to mutually agreeable terms through a formal contract. Unless they are both part-time jobs, you should never sign more than one face sheet at a time, as you are informally committing to two organizations. First, this is ethically questionable, and second, word can get around.

2. Parts of the contract

Contracts are often considered proprietary documents, so although I have pulled out my old contracts to write this section, I have altered details to avoid any issues. This section is a general guide to different parts you should (or might) find in a medical contract and not representative of any one particular document. Also, while certain sections are almost always in the main document, others may be in an "appendix" or "exhibit" at the end of the contract. As long as they show up somewhere in the document, it does not really matter where they are.

Basic information: Most contracts start with some basic information, which may be called "recitals" or "representations." This will list the parties involved – employer, employee (you), and other relevant companies. Physicians are sometimes hired by a physician group or collective that provides services to a hospital rather than directly by the hospital, and this section may clarify that relationship. Practice location(s) should be clearly stated. You need to know which hospitals and clinics you are required to work at on a daily basis or cover when on call. The contract should include a start date and any requirements that need to be completed for the employee to be able to start. This may include items such as completion of hospital credentialing, background check, and proof of immunization. There is usually a term of employment (e.g. 1-3 years), as well as what happens at the end of that term. Many contracts will automatically continue if nothing is done by either party. This needs to be stated, though, so you don't just lose your job at the end of the listed period.

Duties of employee: The contract will list duties of the employee. These generally include regulatory issues, clinical details, and clerical duties. Regulatory issues consist of medical licensure and board certification, completion of continuing medical education requirements (CMEs), application to hospital medical staff and continued medical staff membership, periodic performance review, and ability to practice there (i.e. not restrictively employed somewhere else). Clinical details include required work hours per week and/or weeks per year, call requirements, and providing "high quality" care. I prefer to have specific limits on call in the contract (e.g., "Employee will be required to take 7 days of call per month") rather than less protective statements (e.g., "Call duties will be shared equally among available personnel"). In the second example, if a situation arises where I become the only ENT able to take call, does that mean I have to take call 24/7? That is a scary thought to me. Clerical duties include timely completion of records, attending required organizational meetings, and supervision of other employees. The contract will also state if there is "exclusive employment," meaning you may only work for that company during the contract period and not provide services elsewhere. This usually refers only to employment in your primary medical specialty, but make sure to read the details. If you want to continue your home jewelry-making business, that is generally OK.

Duties of employer: This tells you what the employer is required to do. They are required to compensate you for your work. This may be listed in their duties section or in another area, but you need to know you will get paid. If you are an employed physician rather than in a private practice, the employer is generally responsible for providing personnel and facilities. The contract should state that the employer will supply all personnel needed to do your job. This may include nurses, medical assistants, and a wide variety of clerical staff – billers, office managers, front desk personnel, surgery schedulers, and more. The employer must also provide a physical space for you to work and the necessary medical equipment. This may include medications, medical instruments, surgical tools, scopes, or imaging equipment. The contract should state who determines what is "necessary," and what is done if there is a discrepancy. For example, the employee is sometimes allowed to purchase his/her own equipment if the employer does not deem it necessary. If there is something specific the employer does not already have but you feel it is needed, you can sometimes have that specifically written into your contract. If you need a CO_2 laser for your surgical cases, you might list that in this section (or more likely in an appendix/"exhibit"). The employer is generally responsible for billing the patients and the insurance companies, which is one of the biggest benefits of working for a company rather than owning your own practice. The contract should state this as an employer duty. Finally, the employer should be getting patients for you. I have always worked in places where the supply of patients outweighed the supply of ENT doctors, but if you are in a competitive market, you want to know how your patient supply will be guaranteed.

Compensation: You may be offered a yearly salary, hourly rate, or daily rate. Some positions are payed purely on RVUs (relative value units), but these usually apply after an initial 1-3-year employment period. The contract will state if there is a guaranteed salary, and for how long the salary is guaranteed. There may be exceptions, in that if you do not meet a certain work goal (i.e. less than a certain per cent of the RVU target), the "guaranteed" salary may be reduced. I have never had a problem meeting any of my RVU goals, but you should ask the physicians already in your group how realistic the goals are for that particular practice. You do not want to be in a situation where you are unable to actually make the salary you expect. The RVU target may be explicitly stated (e.g. 6500 RVU per year), or there may be a rate you can calculate (the contract states a guarantee of $350,000 and a rate of $55 per RVU, so you can divide $350,000 by $55 and find that it takes 6364 RVUs to earn your salary). RVU reimbursement rates vary widely by specialty and (hopefully) less widely by institution, so these numbers may be much higher or lower than ones you may see. Any of these models may have bonuses available if you work more than the expected amount. This may be called a productivity bonus or productivity compensation. This may be a dollar amount per RVU, or dollar amount per extra hour or day. The contract should say how frequently these bonuses are calculated (often on a monthly or quarterly basis). There may also be the opposite – that your paycheck is reduced if you do not meet the goal. The contract might mention a salary cap, as well. I recommend being wary of this, as I ran into a problem with it at my first job. The cap was almost twice my base salary, but I reached it within the first 2 years of my employment. The company wanted me to just work for free after reaching the cap, which was not OK with me. In negotiating my next contract, I required the employer to remove the cap so I would not have to worry about it. They were not happy about this, but I felt it was necessary for me to be comfortable with the contract.

Other benefits: Especially if you are working full time, you will often be offered other benefits. These may be listed directly under compensation, or in a separate section. A sign-on bonus is sometimes provided, and/or student loan repayment. Moving reimbursement is another potential benefit. These 3 benefits often have a required employment period. If you do not stay with the employer for the listed amount of time, you may be required to pay back part of all of the amount. Many employers will offer their physicians an annual amount for CME expenses. This can usually be used for conferences, books, and online courses. The employer might reimburse you for licenses or society dues, as well. As an employed physician, you will likely have access to benefits provided to typical employees, like medical, dental, vision, life, and disability insurances. Most larger companies also have retirement plans that can provide tax savings, such as 401(k) or 403(b) products. Some employers also offer a 457(b) for "high-income earners," including physicians. Employers may offer profit sharing or employee contribution matching, as well.

Termination: While we generally hope that we will be happy working at our chosen location for a long time, we need to know the details of how that work agreement might end. It's usually called "termination" in contract lingo, but it's the same as you quitting (termination by employee) or you being fired (termination by employer). This is broken down by "termination for cause" or "termination for convenience." The first means that one of the parties has broken 1 or more of the terms of the contract, and termination is usually quick in this situation (anywhere from immediate to 30 days). Reasons the employer might terminate for cause include that you have failed to uphold the professional standards (e.g. you are showing up drunk to work), you lose your medical license, or you die. The contracts should spell out these reasons. However, the way an employee can terminate for cause sometimes seems more nebulous. If you are considering this and are not sure the employer has violated the contract, you probably need to consult a lawyer. "Termination for convenience" does not need a reason by either party, but usually takes longer. The parties may be required to give from 3 to 6 months notice before actually ending the relationship in this case. This is both so you are not immediately out of job and the company is not immediately without a physician. Once notice has been given, the employer and employee usually work together to set an actual end date and wrap up any ongoing patient care issues. It may be possible to end earlier if both parties agree, and this will usually be stated in the contract.

Non-compete and Non-diversion: Even after you stop working at a company, there may be some restrictions on where or how you can practice. "Non-compete" usually refers to a geographic radius in which you are unable to practice for a certain amount of time after leaving the employer. This is often a 5-30 mile radius for 1-2 years. This may also be called a "restrictive covenant." If nothing like this is listed in your contract, it means this is not a requirement of your employment. You probably want to confirm this with your attorney, but you may not want to specifically mention it to the employer in case it "inspires" them to put it in, which is generally not in your best interest. My first employer specifically told me that they did not have a non-compete because they, "wanted to have doctors available to serve the patients of the area," even if the doctors were not working for them. I have no way of knowing if the rationale is true, but there was no non-compete in the contract. The contract might also discuss "non-diversion" or "non-solicitation." Non-diversion of employees means that you cannot solicit other employees of the company to leave that company and come work with or for you. Non-diversion of patients means that you cannot solicit or encourage your patients or other patients from the organization to follow you to your new position. You can tell patients that you are leaving and they can look you up on their own, but you can't give them your new business card or tell them to come with you if there is a patient non-diversion clause.

Malpractice insurance: This is a big issue in American medicine. Malpractice coverage can be very expensive, so the contract needs to state who is paying for it. All of my employers have paid for my malpractice insurance during the employment period, but I am not sure if this is standard across all specialties or employers. If your employer is not covering it, you need to look up the costs for policies available to you and put this into your budget. Once you finish working for a given company, you need to make sure you are covered for claims that come up after you stop working there. This is most commonly referred to as "tail" insurance coverage. You will sometimes hear about "nose" (or prior acts) insurance coverage. This provides the same coverage as tail insurance, but is offered by the insurer you are joining as opposed to one you are leaving. Either way, many employers will require that you have tail coverage after termination. This is usually a one-time payment of anywhere from $20,000 to $200,000. The contract should state who will pay for it – the employer, the employee, or a percentage for each depending on length of employment. The contract will usually state this, but it is important to understand what is not covered under employer-sponsored malpractice plans. Medical practice outside of your employer – such as moonlighting or medical mission trips – is usually not covered. You will need to obtain alternative coverage for those types of activities. Also, if you commit fraudulent or otherwise criminal acts, you are on your own.

Property: Different types of property may be mentioned, including patient records, confidential company information, and intellectual property. The employer usually retains all rights to the first two types and you are not allowed to disclose any confidential patient or company information. You generally lose access to these records once the agreement is terminated, but there should be a clause that you are given access if needed to defend yourself (e.g. from a malpractice claim). Intellectual property is often addressed in contracts, as well. Each company handles this differently, so make sure you understand how things are written. Some companies say they own all intellectual property you create during your term of employment, even if it was done on your own time using only your own resources. Others say that you get it all and they get nothing. Many are in the middle, saying you retain rights as long as you are not doing it at work, on company time, or with company equipment. Some require you to notify them before starting anything in order to protect your personal claim to the intellectual property. Again, this may be negotiable if it is important to you.

Limit on outside activities: Contracts may limit some of your activities while you are employed with the company. The most common thing I see is limits on working in the medical field at other locations during hours you are not scheduled to work at your primary job (a.k.a. "moonlighting"). They probably do not care if you want to work a few hours at Starbucks. You can generally volunteer anywhere you want, but there are often limits in using your affiliation with your employer. For example, if you offer to give a medical talk for free, you may be required to put the company logo on your slides, have your slides approved, or not mention the company in any way. You may be prohibited from accepting honoraria or travel funds, or required to turn such monies over to the employer. As a reminder, volunteering your medical service (e.g. mission trips, "team doctor" for school sports) is often not covered by employer-sponsored malpractice insurance, so make sure to check on that. Some organizations have a "code of conduct" in which you are supposed to be an upstanding individual and represent yourself well in your community. Does this mean you can't get drunk at a bar with your friends? You're probably fine, as long as you're not saying bad things about your company. We've all heard about medical professionals who have lost their jobs from Facebook posts that were in bad taste, though, so just be careful.

Buy-in: If you are signing a contract with a private practice rather than a hospital, there may be information about "buy-in." This means that after a certain amount of time, you have the opportunity to purchase a part of the practice, so you become a business owner instead of an employee. This section should include the length of time you have to work there before you are eligible for the buy-in, as well as an expiration for the buy-in. It should also include what happens if you choose not to buy in. Can you continue to work there under the same contract terms, or do you have to find a new job? There may be certain work conditions you have to meet to be eligible, as well. For example, you may have to meet certain RVU targets, patient satisfaction or other survey goals, or pass some sort of vote by the current owners. It is best when these conditions are objective to save you the nightmare of being "voted out" even though you have served your time there. (That being said, you probably don't want to buy into a practice where the people are a bunch of jerks!) The contract should list the cost of the buy-in, either as a dollar figure or a percent of some value (i.e. estimated business net worth, revenue or profits in the past year). If an actual number is not given, it is appropriate to ask so you can financially plan for the amount of money you need to save.

Changes: Contracts often have sections discussing the policy on changes that happen after a contract is signed. These include changes in employer policies and external laws. Generally, if an external law changes, both employee and employer are required to follow the new law. However, if the employer changes one of its policies, what are your options? If you disagree with the change, are you allowed to terminate for cause? If this section is not in the contract, I would not worry about it too much unless you hear in your interview about any major changes coming. This is sometimes the case when one hospital or health system is bought out by another.

Arbitration: If the employer and employee have a disagreement, there has to be a way to settle it. Many contracts state that matters will be settled by arbitration. This is not the same as a regular court hearing, in that there is no right to appeal the decision. Judge and jury are also absent. An arbitrator is supposed to be neutral, but arbitration is usually set in the city or county where the employer is located. If you have a powerful employer, I am not sure how neutral the arbitration might be. However, this may be one of the few things that you can't really negotiate. So just make sure your contract is written well so you don't have to deal with the arbitration!

Reference to other materials: To make them more confusing, contracts often refer to other sections within the contract or "exhibits" attached to the contract. This information will usually be given to you all at once. However, contracts will often mention other external documents. These may include hospital bylaws, employee handbooks, or state laws. If the employer does not automatically provide these documents for you, you should request them from the employer so you know what you are agreeing to. I would not recommend signing the contract until you receive and review these documents.

3. Other contracts

The information above focuses on contracts where you are a physician hired by a hospital, practice, or group. If you are self-employed or looking at a partnership contract, there will likely be a lot of different information. Talk to a lawyer and/or use available online resources. If you are working as an independent contractor, like with most locum tenens situations, the contracts may be much simpler. There is usually a several page general contract between you and the locum company itself. This will spell out some of the items listed above, such as contract term and termination, duties of each party, and malpractice. Since you are usually an independent contractor rather than an employee, the contract will usually state that fact and the details around it (i.e. that you do not receive classic benefits, and you are usually responsible for making your own tax payments). There is also a "face sheet" for each assignment that spells out the pay rates and specific duties of that assignment. These simpler contracts were a breath of fresh air for me after dealing with 4 months of negotiations over a 50-page contract, but I did make a lot more money at my employed positions.

4. Contract negotiation

Yes, negotiations are often frustrating. Hopefully you don't have to do it too often. You do get better at it over time, too. I did not have any sort of guide like this the first (or even the second) time I negotiated medical contracts. It would have been extremely helpful, so I hope it helps take some of the stress and confusion away from your experience.

First thing to realize: Everything is negotiable, even the things people tell you are not negotiable. There are usually at least a few small things you will want to have changed, but there can sometimes be major issues. Contracts may be missing important pieces, or may contradict what you were told during your interview. The contract is the legal document that binds you and the employer, so you need to make sure it is right. Any "promises" not in the contract do not have to be followed, so make sure you get everything important in writing. You don't want to come across as a jerk, but it's better to be a stickler than to sign something you're not comfortable with.

Be prepared to know of any "walk away" conditions you might have. For example, if you are absolutely not willing to take more than 2 weeks of call per month and the contract does not protect you from this, it might not be the right company for you. Like I said, everything is negotiable, but the company (or you) might not be willing to make certain concessions. I had some major problems with my first contract, and I was absolutely unwilling to sign another contract with the same problems. Sticking to my guns could have cost me a job (especially if it had been a more competitive market), but the company and I were eventually able to negotiate an agreement that was acceptable to both parties. I went into negotiations knowing what conditions would make me walk away, and I ended up with a good contract because of it. That being said, don't lose a good job because of stubbornness. But *do* walk away from a job offer if you know it's not right for you.

You will want to make a list of all of the items you would like to change in the contract. You should have this grouped for yourself as "optional items" and "necessary items." The "necessary items" are your walk away points, whereas optional ones are just things you would like but don't actually need. You may also want to separate minor versus major changes. For example, a minor change may be a change in wording that your lawyer suggested to make sure something is clear. A major change would be something like the tail coverage structure or call duties.

How do you decide what you need or want to negotiate? The section above that talks about the parts of the contract should be helpful, but every individual has his or her own priorities. I was not comfortable agreeing to call that my partners were not required to take, but that might not have been an issue for some people.

Others might worry about salary a lot more than I did. This is a time when you really need to ask yourself what is important to you (and potentially your spouse or dependents) and use that as your guide. You generally don't want to argue every single item in the contract, but if something is important to you, definitely bring it up. Once you sign the contract, it's very hard to make changes later.

There are various strategies on how to present your points:
Strategy #1: List the most important things first, and funnel down to least important at the end.
Strategy #2: Give the other party a couple items at a time, then once those are addressed, submit the next few things.
Strategy #3: Come up with more things than you actually care about, present them all, and see which ones are accepted (i.e. "swing for the fences").
Strategy #4: List all items in the order they come up in the contract.

I prefer strategy #4. Especially when you have documents over 50 pages long, it is easiest just to go in order rather than jumping all over the place. In a sort of "gamesmanship" strategy, I like this method since it gets everything out on the table without necessarily revealing your hand. You and the company may have very different ideas of what is important. You may request something you think is a big deal, only to have them agree to it right away. It may be that you are hiring on with the greatest company in the world, but there are some companies who will try to leverage you if they know what is most important to you.

If you use strategy #1 with presenting the most important items first, it can be tough if your employer doesn't agree with them. However, if they've decided they're only going to agree to 3 things, you at least have gotten your 3 most important ones doing it this way. I don't like strategy #2 because it reminds me of a horrible experience my husband and I had with a mortgage officer. She would ask for documents and we would provide them, but then she would keep asking for a few more documents in each of her subsequent e-mails. This drove me insane. I just wanted her to tell us everything she needed so we could take care of it all at once (rather than her continuing to request things when our papers were eventually packed into a storage locker in another state!). But I digress. Strategy #3 might overwhelm the employer if you end up with a lot of requests, but if the employer goes into negotiations saying they'll only accept 50% of your suggestions, this will get you the most (of course you don't know the employer's mindset, though). You can use whatever strategy you like, but you want to think about what you are doing.

It will usually take several – or many – exchanges to get all of your points addressed. Items that the other party thinks are trivial will often be agreed to right away. They may state that they need to take certain issues to their legal team. Your main e-mail point of contact is sometimes an actual decision maker, but other times is more of a go-between. I have had situations where this contact person has said that a request was "non-negotiable," so I have had to go up the chain of command. Each time this has happened, I have been given contact information for a more senior person and gotten my needs addressed. Most negotiations these days are done via e-mail, but you may need or want to talk to someone on the phone if e-mail is not accomplishing your goal.

One thing to consider in contract negotiations is any equipment or personnel that you need or want. There is not usually a section for this in the contract, so this would likely be an addendum. For example, one condition of your employment might be that the hospital purchases nerve monitoring equipment that you (and likely other surgeons) can use for certain cases. If it is in the contract and they don't purchase it, you can hold them in breach of contract. If it's not in the contract but they said they would buy it, they are not legally obligated to do so and you might be out of luck. You don't want to overwhelm them with requests, but you need to make sure you'll have what you need to do your job.

So what items do you actually negotiate? The easy answer is, 'Whatever matters to you.' This could be salary, call, benefits, salary cap, or anything else you can think of, whether or not it is listed in the prior sections. You should be realistic in your negotiations, though. If you want them to pay you $500k starting salary but it is your first year out of residency and the median starting salary in your field is $200k, that's probably not going to work. If you worked very hard at your current job and were in the 95th percentile of earners in your field, though, you may be able to negotiate a higher salary at the next job than what is initially being offered. It is very helpful to have numbers and experience to support your requests.

In addition to things that you want, you really need to negotiate any terms in the contract that may be unfavorable to you. This could be a prohibitive salary cap, an overly-restrictive non-compete, or termination conditions. For example, if you as the employee terminate for cause (meaning the employer violated a term of the contract), you should not be required to pay back the signing bonus. There is often a minimum employment term to avoid paying back all or a portion of moving expenses, student loan repayment, signing bonuses, and sometimes tail malpractice coverage. These terms generally should not apply if you terminate for cause or the employer terminates for convenience. This needs to be spelled out in the contract. Also, if things are poorly or unclearly worded, minor changes can often be made. This is one of the parts where the lawyer is most helpful, as he or she is much more used to reading legal documents.

SECTION THREE: Doing the Job

You're hired! Great news. You're finally starting your career. The first step will be the (generally painful) process of hospital credentialing, where you have to fill out a lot of paperwork to make sure you are qualified to work there and that the hospital will get paid for you seeing patients. This can take several months, so even if you've started your job search early, it may be time for a much needed vacation. Plus once you've signed a long-term contract, who knows the next time you can take more than a week or two off at a time.

As with most things in life, better results usually come with effort and planning. You've spent many years learning how to take care of patients. This section probably takes less than two hours to read, but will guide you in how to take care of your career. Some of us get bits and pieces of this information in residency lectures or from colleagues, but I've tried to put together the relevant information in one place.

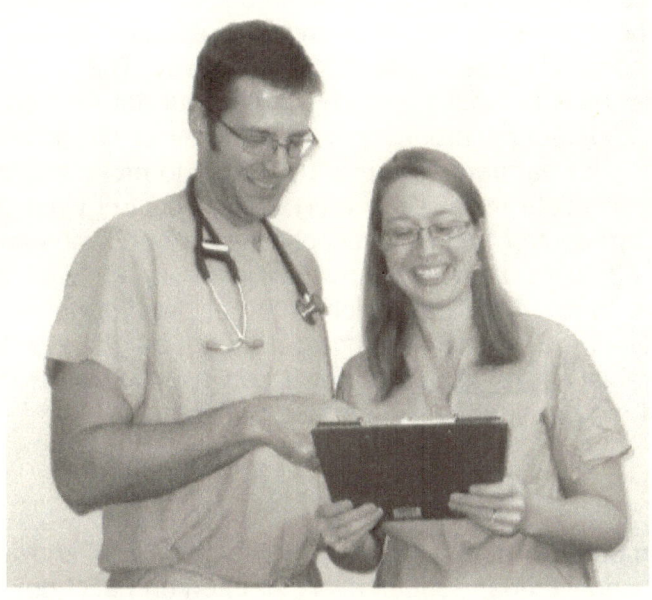

Cover photo from my prior book:
Two "doctors" doing their jobs

Chapter One: Taking Care of Yourself

As physicians, our job is to take care of other people. However, we cannot do this if we do not take care of ourselves first. I felt that the ability to truly care for myself was very limited in residency, but I have made it a priority out in practice. I strongly recommend that you do, too. Not only will it make you a happier person, but it will make you a better doctor. If we are filled with stress, we cannot truly care for our patients.

If you're in a situation that is making you miserable, you essentially have four choices:

1. Accept the situation.
2. Change the situation.
3. Change your response.
4. Walk away.

I don't recommend option #1, as you'll still be miserable. However, it seems like this is what a lot of people do with their lives. They just accept the frustrating job, the uncaring spouse, or the horrible neighborhood. Life doesn't have to be this way! The second option is great when it is feasible. Have the hospital get new equipment, change the personnel around you, or lighten your call schedule with help from your partners. If you are not able to make any changes, though, you might try #3. You can't always control what happens, but you can control how you respond. In residency, it seemed like #1 and #3 were really the only options, so #3 was definitely preferable to #1. The final option is to get out. I'm not advocating you quit your job whenever things get tough, but you don't want to be miserable the rest of your life. If options #1-3 aren't cutting it, option #4 may be your only chance to be happy.

1. Get Help if You Need It

Physician suicide rates are disturbingly high. We all know this is a problem, and we hear about it every so often on Facebook or in the news. You may think, "This could never happen to me or someone I care about," and hopefully you're right. However, you need to recognize the warning signs in yourself so you can take action before it even gets close. Thankfully, most people don't take the furthest extreme of suicide, but there are many more people who are depressed or are miserable at their jobs. I've had a number of patients over the years who have been visibly distraught in office visits or said things that I just can't ignore. Even as an ENT surgeon, sometimes talking about a patient's recurrent tonsillitis is not the most important thing, and I need to address his emotions. I try to make sure they're safe, and then contact the PCP so we can find some resources to help. When I was in a situation where I was miserable with my job, it took me a while to figure out exactly what to do. A patient only has to cry once for me to say something. I was crying almost every day without doing anything about it for a while. Why are we more caring towards our patients than we are towards ourselves?

As physicians – and I think especially surgeons – we are used to being able to take care of problems on our own. In a surgical residency, you are "weak" if you cry or get upset, and you need to get things done without "excuses." (Personally, I didn't feel like it was an excuse when I couldn't study for the next day's case when I had been up all night taking care of critically ill patients, but my attending disagreed.) This culture needs to change. Since we can only control our own behavior, the change starts by being nicer to ourselves and others and being more aware of what's going on. It takes strength to admit that something is wrong. We have all learned the symptoms of depression, but it's worth listing some of them again:

– Losing interest in activities, hobbies, or socializing
– Feeling hopeless
– Sleep disturbance
– Repeatedly getting angry or irritated by minor issues
– Using illegal substances
– Using legal substances in a harmful way (too much or too little food, improper use of prescription medications, overuse of alcohol)
– Making plans or attempting to hurt yourself

Every hospital I have worked at has had resources for physicians to deal with mental health issues. They are usually brought up during your benefits overview or can be found on the organizational website. There's often something called the "employee assistance plan," and it has free anonymous counselors. There are also many internet and phone resources available through a Google search. While talking to a trusted friend or family member may be a good starting point, that person may not have the expertise you need to get the right help.

2. Get Help Even if You Think You Don't Need It

None of us should have to go through life alone. There is always a colleague, friend, family member, religious leader, or counselor that can help you with a problem you might be facing. Bad things are going to happen at times, and even if we are not dealing with depression, drug abuse, or suicide, we can still use help from others. Your relationships with others will be much deeper and more meaningful if you share both the good and the bad.

My husband heard me complain about residency all the time. When I got together with work friends at my first job out of residency, most of what we did was complain and gossip about work. I don't think I was being a negative person or a whiner, but I needed to vent my frustrations. Even now that my work situation has improved, I still talk to colleagues when I have a challenging case or a bad outcome, and to my friends and family if there are other problems. Some people prefer to express their emotions in a journal or with poetry or song, but we all need some sort of outlet. However you choose to get help, don't let problems build to the point where things cannot be undone.

Where does physician burnout fit in? It's a serious problem that affects many physicians to varying degrees. I definitely dealt with burnout at one of my jobs after residency. Talking to my husband and colleagues was helpful for dealing with the emotional aspect, but they could not fix the problem. I expressed my concerns to the organization, and they did not support me in finding any solutions. I eventually had to leave the organization. Quitting the job, taking time off, thinking about my priorities, and changing my work schedule at my next job all helped, but it was a rough time. If your organization can't or won't help you, I would recommend taking some time off to consider your options. It's nearly impossible to deal with burnout when you keep going to the same job every day.

3. Handling Stress

Even if physicians don't want to admit we have "problems" as in #2, I think we all admit that we deal with stress. The nature of the job itself is stressful since we are dealing with life and death situations with patients. We are often asked to do more than we can find the time or energy to accomplish. We need to recognize stress and learn to manage it.

The first step is to identify our stressors. This can include issues both at work and at home. You may want someone to help you with this, because it's sometimes hard to see when we are caught up in the middle of things. Just promise that person not to take out your stress on them! The second is to try to eliminate or reduce any stressors we have control over. If you are always worried about what you are going to make for dinner after work, make a meal plan ahead of time, cook over the weekend for the rest of the week, or have someone else take over meals (whether it's a spouse, family member, friend, or someone you hire). Finances are a huge source of stress for many people, but often don't have to be. Section Four of this book should help a lot with that. The third step is to address the stressors over which we have very little control. As an employed physician, I usually do not get to choose the people I work with. However, I can choose how I react to them. If there's a bad situation, I can document what is happening and report it up the chain of command. If I have tried to talk to people within an organization and feel like I have exhausted all available channels, my only options may be changing my reaction or getting out of the situation altogether. Again, I am not advocating quitting your job whenever things get tough, but it sometimes seems the only way to protect yourself.

In addition to identifying and dealing with specific stressors, general stress reduction techniques are often beneficial. I once tried "mindfulness meditation" and couldn't stand it. I just kept thinking, "I could be doing so many productive things with this time rather than sitting here trying to think of nothing." Clearly, there is not one strategy that works for everyone. Although in my first book I said that exercise was not helpful for me, I have revised that now. I think when you are extremely sleep deprived and exhausted at baseline, exercise may not have the same psychological or physiological benefits it has for the "normal" person. I think that rather than encouraging everyone to exercise, we should encourage people to take care of themselves physically to help themselves mentally. My body (and brain) needed sleep as a resident. Now that I get enough sleep, it does feel good to stretch and be active, whether it's taking a walk or doing a 45-minute cardio workout. Meditation or yoga work well for certain individuals. Some people have mental scripts for decreasing stress, or work through a head-to-toe relaxation exercise. Others turn to professionals, either for counseling or medication. There is no single right way. You just need to find what works for you and do it.

4. Work/Life Balance

In organizing this chapter, I started off with the "worst" and moved on to the "best." A lot of people throw around "work/life balance" as a catch phrase that the "young physicians" care about and the "older generation" doesn't really think about, but it's much more than that. It's about combining your career and your life outside of work in a way that makes you productive and happy in both arenas. You have to choose how much time and energy you devote to each part, as time and energy are both limited resources. As we know, we're more effective at our jobs if we're happy. Work/Life Balance is how we get to achieve that happiness.

A lot of us find joy in our jobs, and hopefully in our life outside work, too. (I know I do!) We deal with stress and problems in both of these arenas, as well. As physicians, we need to find a balance between our time at work and at home so we can be successful in both. When things are going badly at home, we want there to be something positive we can focus on at work to help us make it through. Our friends and family members help us endure tough times at work. When we're choosing a job or making life plans, we need to think about how our choices will let us accomplish this. If a job requires you to be on call the same time as your physician spouse, how are you going to care for your children? Do you get a nanny or help from family, or is it best not to accept that particular job? If you really enjoy your hobby of competitive cycling and are already feeling pressed for time, do you want to accept the promotion to assistant department chair? Do you want to marry the person you're dating even though he lives in another city and you'd have to find a new job, or do you keep the job you currently love? None of these are easy choices, but they are choices we face, and should think about in the context of work/life balance.

In addition to these fairly recognizable choices, a lot of the challenges in striking a good work/life balance are insidious. More and more obligations get added at work to the point where you realize you're working 70 hours a week instead of 50. Or your kids get older, and each one has picked up an additional extra-curricular activity over the past couple years, so the schedules conflict so much you can't physically attend every activity. This type of situation is much easier to prevent than it is to address once it has happened. The key is learning to say no. Most of us want to be helpful, but we can't do that to the extent of sacrificing ourselves. I have felt that some employers will try to squeeze everything they can out of me, and they often do not care about the results. I have gotten a lot better at saying no over the years. At home, you may have to prioritize your own hobbies to make time for the ones that are most important to you. Maybe you can bake something for the PTA, but you can't commit to being on their board.

Even if you are single or childless, you deserve work/life balance. Just because your colleague decided to have 5 kids does not make his time more valuable than yours. You should not have to stay later at the office just because you don't have kids. You may have chosen to be single at this point so you don't have as many factors to include in the work/life balance equation. Then you can choose if you want to spend more time becoming the world expert on Kawasaki disease, or traveling the world in your time off.

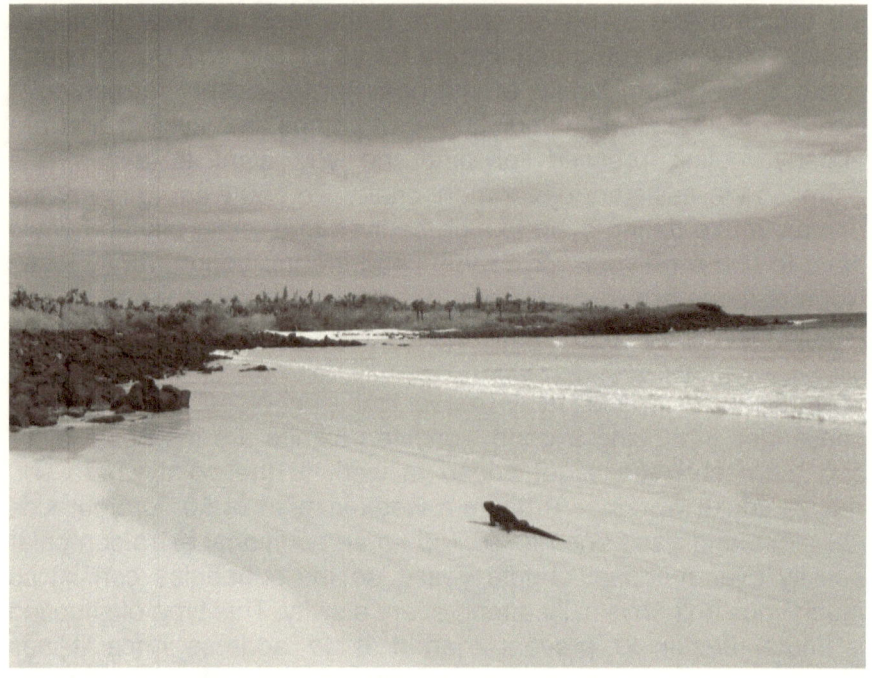
Traveling the world: A marine iguana in the Galapagos

Chapter Two: Scheduling

You will usually have some control over how your workday or week is scheduled. The main concepts here are schedule templates, block time, and time off. If you do straight shift work, some of this will not apply. However, you may still have designated administrative time that is nice to schedule to your advantage.

1. Schedule templates

If you work in an outpatient clinic, your patients will generally have appointment times. Some clinics run on a model where there are no appointments and they see as many people as they have time for, but this is not as common in my experience. As a patient, I prefer to have a set appointment time. As an ENT doctor, I want to make sure I can see my patient with throat cancer when he shows up rather than my patient with tonsil stones even if the cancer patient showed up later in the day. The clinics that run without appointments are often seeing indigent patients and/or the supply of patients severely outweighs the supply of physicians. You might have the option to choose either model, but it is often predetermined for you.

You may or may not have some leeway in your appointment times. Places I have worked schedule either 20 or 30 minutes for a new patient, and generally 15 minutes for a follow-up or post-op visit. The first week or two at a new place, they usually give you longer visits to get used to the system, but you are quickly ramped up to full speed. Certain specialties may have longer or shorter appointment times. You can usually request individual patients to be scheduled in certain ways, too. For example, if you have a patient you see every 3 months to clean her ears and you know it takes 30 minutes each time, you can usually have your schedulers block 30 instead of 15 minutes. Your clinic may not give you much flexibility in the general appointment times, but if you are always running behind, the patients and staff will be unhappy, so something will have to change. Hopefully they won't just tell you you have to speed up.

If there are different types of visits (e.g. new patients, follow-ups, post-ops), you can either build your template so the schedulers put any patient at any time, or schedule different visit types at different times. For example, you might have your first 2 visits of the day as new patients, then 3 follow ups, then 3 new patients, 2 post-ops, and then lunch. Scheduling this way is a little more complex to set up at first, but it does make sure you are reserving spots for different patient types. If your clinic is really busy and you don't have any time set aside, your schedule might be filled with new patients so you don't have time to see your post-op or follow-up patients.

2. Block time

If you are a surgeon, you or your group will be given OR block time. You may be working at multiple ORs, often including hospitals and surgery centers. For example, I might be given every Thursday at the surgery center and every other Monday at the hospital OR. You usually do not get to choose when your block time is, so if this is very important to you, find out about it in your interview and get it into your contract. Some hospitals have plenty of block time to go around, but it is hard to get at others. Surgeons need to ask about this in the interview. Sometimes the block time is for your practice, and you and your partners share it. Again, you need to know how much you will get.

It is also important to know about policies regarding block time. If you end up needing more than what is allotted, what is the process? Are you only able to pick up available random time (i.e., when other surgeons go on vacation and their time becomes available), or can you somehow get more? Also, there is a risk of losing your reserved block time if you are not using enough of it. You should know the policies on this at your hospital, and talk to your surgery scheduler and/or surgical scheduling department if you are at risk.

3. Time off

Time away from work generally has to be scheduled in advance. For most jobs, you will be given a certain amount of time off per year. This may be separated out into vacation, CME, sick days, and holidays, or it may be all combined into a total amount of time off. As soon as you know of dates you want off, talk to your partners to make sure patient care needs will be covered. Someone is usually needed to cover call, and some practices have policies that at least 50% of the physicians in the group have to be present at all times (or something similar).

Some practices also give you "administrative time." This is time to catch up on paperwork, attend meetings, or address other patient-related tasks while you are not actually scheduled to be seeing patients. You may be required to be in the office during your admin time, or you may be able to do other things as long as you put in the hours at some other point. For example, when I worked part time at a job 5 hours from my home, I would take my admin time Friday afternoons and start my drive home as soon as I finished seeing patients. Then I would spend a few hours on the weekend finishing notes and doing my other administrative duties. Other colleagues have worked their admin time around children's schedules or personal appointments if they do not have required meetings at work. The downside to admin time is that if you're paid purely on an RVU basis, you are not doing billable work during your admin time, so it decreases your productivity and therefore your salary.

Chapter Three: Electronic Medical Record

Most practices now have an EMR, or electronic medical record. It goes by other acronyms, such as EHR (electronic health record) or CPOE (computerized physician order entry). The EMR is helpful in many ways – accessing records from other doctors and departments, avoiding illegible handwriting and handwriting errors, providing many interaction warnings on medications and allergies, and assisting in order entry. However, it is often a huge time sink, can create errors of its own, and (like any computer program) sometimes crashes. You want to become at least moderately savvy with your hospital's EMR so you can be as efficient as possible. Although the EMR has benefits, we know it can use up an inordinate amount of time. Try to waste as little time as possible here!

1. EMR Training

Whenever you start a new job, you usually have to do some sort of EMR training. This may be as short as an hour or extend over 1-2 weeks. The smarter organizations take into account your pre-existing experience with EMRs in general and their particular EMR, but others make all new employees do the same training. The problem with most training programs (other than the fact that they are redundant and mind-numbing) is that they have limited relevance to what you might be doing. All of the places I have been trained have directed the training at inpatient hospitalists. So if you are an inpatient hospitalist, the training might actually be helpful for you. But for everyone else, you will need to learn a lot of what you actually need to know from the other physicians doing the same or similar work.

The trainer may be able to customize some settings for you. If you have already used that organization's particular EMR or are familiar with similar ones, you may know what you want right away. Otherwise, it is helpful to meet with the trainer again after you have been there for a week or two to have them customize once you see what actually works for you. Some trainers may be able to sit with you when you are first seeing patients to help you as you go along.

If you have created any EMR shortcut phrases in residency or at another job, save them. You may be able to upload them to your new system, or have the IT people do it for you.

2. EMR Efficiency

Although EMRs can be helpful in many ways, I have not found any of them to be inherently efficient in writing notes. There is either a lot of typing or clicking in any default set up. You will spend a VERY LONG time writing notes if you do not make some shortcuts. Some people use templated notes for a certain visit type (e.g. new patient with diabetes or post-op appendectomy). These can be for inpatient, outpatient, or emergency room visits. Depending on what you need to document (see later coding chapter for details), you may want to have many different notes that are pre-tailored, or have a few broad notes to which you may quickly add details. You may build personal or institutional shortcuts into these notes, which will save you additional time. These can automatically pull in patient history information, vital signs, and review of systems data. Some people prefer to use notes built by the institution or EMR and click on boxes that show if a symptom is present or absent or if an exam finding is normal or abnormal. These are not efficient for me personally, but they might work for you.

In addition to entire notes, most EMRs will let you create shortcuts for words or phrases of any length. Each EMR will have different names for these items, like "short keys," "smart lists," or "dot phrases." EMR trainers like to use their specific terminology, but the ideas are all similar. In most cases, you can pull from some that were created by other users or by the system, as well as make your own. In addition to text, you can use these links to pull in data such as recent labs, vital signs for a given amount of time, or radiology results. Ask your EMR trainer for a list of such phrases at your institution. Pre-built lists are often available for common choices, and can sometimes be created for you. You may have lists for times (e.g. follow up in "x days, weeks, or months"), symptoms (pain described as "burning, shooting, stabbing, throbbing"), people (history provided by "patient, mother, father, daughter, guardian"), or anything else you can think of.

Dictation can be combined with most EMRs. Dragon is an instant talk to text dictation that is very popular. It is most helpful for things that are different for different patients, such as HPI (history of present illness) and certain treatment plans. If something is the same every time, use the above templates so you can fill it in with a couple keystrokes rather than having to recite the same paragraph over and over. Other systems have you place a marker within a note to show where a dictation should go, and you then dictate to a transcription service where another person types what you have said after the fact. This situation takes longer for the notes to be finalized, but might save you time overall.

You also want to learn where things are located in your EMR – radiology links to images, pathology reports, previous notes, patient contact information, and anything else you may want to look up. You might have medical assistants who will try to find this information for you and potentially even include it in your note, but you need to know how to access it yourself, as well. There will be times when you need the information and your go-to medical assistant is not available.

In an ideal world, your schedule would work out where you can look up your patient, see your patient, and complete your documentation on that patient during that patient's scheduled visit. Patients would not get confused in your memory because you would only be dealing with one patient at a time. You would only look up a lab result or pull up images once, because you would document the results immediately. This would clearly be the most efficient way to do things. However, this usually does not happen for me. A patient shows up late, or it takes longer to explain things to them, or there are multiple issues to address in a given visit, or you end up needing to do a procedure, or you get pulled away by a page or a consult. Then you are left completing your notes during your lunch "break" or at the end of the day after seeing all of your patients. You don't remember the discharge plan from the recent hospitalization, or how many positive strep tests the patient had in the past year, and you have to look it up again. It's also possible to forget exactly what you said or did in the encounter.

I have a few strategies I use to address this reality. When I am taking the history in the exam room, I usually type while the patient is talking. I make sure I have at least partial eye contact with the patient during this time so they still feel I am focused on them. There are times when I need to stop typing depending on what is happening with the patient, but I am usually able to get most of the HPI in while the patient is talking. Then I might use the EMR to pull up images to show the patient, and also to order medications or tests at the end of the visit. Sometimes you need to enter the follow-up information while the patient is still in the room so the check-out desk knows what to do when the patient leaves. If I do not have time to finish the entire note, I try to at least document any abnormalities in the exam before I move on to the next patient. Although it is less efficient, I can usually remember and piece together enough information from the rest of the note and orders to document my medical decision making when I get back to the notes later on. I do not like to keep my patients waiting, so if I am running behind, I sacrifice some efficiency for patient satisfaction.

3. EMR Accuracy

With all of the above shortcuts, you need to make sure your EMR documentation is accurate. If you deviate from your standard for some reason, you need to make sure you document that. Automatic signatures and time stamps are common with EMRs, so if you are documenting something after the fact, make sure you note when the service actually took place and why it is late if there is a time-sensitive situation. You also want to proofread anything that is dictated or free-typed to make sure there are no significant typographical errors. If you notice a mistake after you have already signed a note, you will generally need to do an addendum to correct it. Finally, you need to make sure your EMR is accurate in capturing what you have actually done. This will be further discussed with the coding chapter.

Chapter Four: Medical Coding

Unfortunately, the medical system has invented an arcane way compute a value for each task we do as physicians. So do you pull out your hair and scream? No! Use your knowledge of the system to your advantage. If you know how to properly code, it will help you get paid for what you're already doing. We are not "gaming the system" by accurately documenting what we do. In fact, we are improving our communication by writing good notes, protecting ourselves from malpractice suits, and avoiding fraud.

** READ THE NEXT THREE PARAGRAPHS EVEN IF YOU THINK YOU DO NOT NEED TO KNOW ANYTHING ABOUT CODING. **

You might not care about coding, but you should. At many jobs, it determines how much you get paid. This is if your payment or bonuses are based on RVUs. Sometimes it can help justify hiring additional staff. (One of the places I worked said that they could not hire an extra medical assistant for us because the medical assistant to physician ratio was tied into the department RVUs.) Finally, doing it correctly will help you avoid an audit or fraud.

Some physicians are responsible for entering the final numeric code, or for doing coding using "descriptive words." If you're using the numeric codes, you need to know how you're choosing those numbers. If you are using the "descriptive words," you need to read this chapter or at least the CMS guidelines (links at the end of the text) to figure out what the descriptive words mean. Spoiler alert: They do not mean what you think they mean.

You might be in the increasingly rare group of physicians who say, "Oh, I don't have to know this at all, since I have coders that do this for me." Well, you know what? Even if you don't have to enter any part of the code (numbers or descriptions), your coders are using the information in this section to determine the codes. The codes that they determine may be determining your salary. So making small changes in your documentation may make big changes in your paycheck. For the people in this (small) group, don't worry about adding the points and determining levels. *Do* look at what types of documentation lead to each code.

Although this is kind of a long section, it is really just an introduction to coding. A lot of resources are available online, and there are coding courses and workshops you can attend. For example, there is an ENT coding workshop offered every year at our ENT Academy annual meeting, and it is quite popular. Some employers have coding specialists that work with physicians, as well. One of my employers had a one-on-one coding session for me as part of the initial orientation process, so that was quite nice. Sometimes employers have coders that periodically review your charts and tell you what you've done wrong with coding. This can be helpful, too, but is usually not "fun." The main advantage to employer-based coding support is that it is free for you. However, the coder probably is not an expert in your specialty. You generally have to pay for the off-site workshops, but it can be worth it as you may greatly increase your revenue by improving your coding and documentation.

1. Step back: Documentation

I called this chapter "coding," because the idea is to teach you proper coding. However, the real underlying goal is to correctly document what you do. In an ideal world, you would just do what you need to do to take care of your patient, and you would be paid for it. In the real world, though, this doesn't work. If I do sinus surgery for a patient, I get paid based on *what I document*. If I am asked to see a patient for a neck mass, the complexity of the interaction is determined by *what I document* about the history I take, the exam I perform, and the medical decision making that is involved (more on all these later). As you've probably heard before, "If it isn't documented, it wasn't done." Even if you did a lot of work, if you don't document it properly, you won't get credit for it. Gone are the days of getting paid for hand writing something like, "AOM. Abx." (Translation: Patient has acute otitis media. Will treat with antibiotics.)

In addition to allowing for accurate coding, you want your documentation to facilitate communication with other medical personnel. It is often important for other people to know what you did or found for a given patient. If the hospitalist Dr. Tran asked you to consult on her inpatient Mrs. Carlisle, you should specifically let Dr. Tran know your findings and recommendations. However, Mrs. Carlisle's primary doctor, a different specialist, and any covering physicians may also want to know what you did. You probably don't want each person to call or page you for that information, so you should write it down in a clear way.

Speaking of clarity in documentation, most hospital systems now have electronic medical records. This has really helped with the illegible handwriting problem, but we are still plagued with TLAs – three letter acronyms. Some of these TLAs are so common across all fields of medicine that they probably won't cause a second thought. I don't think many physicians have to think about the meaning of HTN. However, some mean different things to different people. To me as an ENT, BMT means bilateral myringotomy with tubes. However, to a hematologist, BMT is more likely to mean bone marrow transplant. It's kind of important to know which of these procedures we are considering! Other TLAs may be known only to you or the people at your training program. A vascular surgeon told me he kept reading "VLB" in notes from his PA. He had no idea what it was, so finally asked. Apparently the PA used it for vascular lab, but the surgeon who worked right along with him had no clue. I frequently read notes from other doctors and am unclear on their acronyms. Question: Do I personally use them? Of course! But I try to make sure that the main communication sections of my note – i.e. the assessment and plan – have very limited abbreviations, or that I have put the full term in parenthesis. For example, I might write, "SMG (submandibular gland)" at the beginning of the assessment, and then just use "SMG" throughout the rest of the section. Many EMRs allow you to set up short cuts for some of these abbreviations so you can just type "SNHL" but "sensorineural hearing loss" will actually display in the note.

Along with avoiding abbreviations, explaining your thought process is always a good idea. This doesn't necessarily mean you need to write long paragraphs, but you want anyone looking at the note to know what you were thinking. If you see a patient with hearing loss and your plan is to order a hearing test, that doesn't really need a lot of explanation. However, if you are seeing a patient who has severe hypertension and you are NOT starting them on an antihypertensive medication, you probably ought to say why. You always want to document *what* you are doing, but a good guideline is to make sure you also explain *why* you are doing something if it deviates from standard practice. This helps you and your colleagues understand your rationale, and can also help protect you in potential malpractice situations. I've read many notes where people did not document what or why. The doctors writing these notes may be wonderful clinicians and people, but if I can't understand it, it's not helpful for our shared patient. Knowing what I do about coding makes me wonder how they're actually getting paid with such poor documentation, as well.

The note structure itself can help or hinder electronic communication. We are traditionally taught the SOAP note in med school – subjective, objective, assessment, plan. This generally reflects the order in which the information flows, but does not put the most important information at the top of the note. I have heard some people promote the APSO note instead, where you put the assessment and plan right at the top. I have not seen many people actually adopt it, so I have trained myself to almost immediately scroll down to the bottom of other doctors' notes that I read. Although I still follow the SOAP note order, I try to reduce redundancy. Many EMR notes have full lists of past medical history, medications, labs, and imaging reports pulled into the note text. This is a lot to scroll through. I put in my notes a statement that those items have been reviewed, and only provide the relevant information directly in the body of my note. (I'll include an explanation/example later to show how to do this and still get proper credit for it.) This makes my notes shorter and avoids redundancy. I feel like it actually makes it easier to concentrate while reading the note, as people tend to zone out more the longer a list gets.

In addition to being accurate and understandable, documentation should be done in a timely fashion. First off, it's a lot easier to remember what you saw and did if you write it down right away. I discussed in the EMR efficiency section how I do my notes. I make sure to finish all of them within 24 hours, and preferably before I go home for the evening. In some situations, it's very important to patient care to enter documentation even sooner. For example, I saw 2 patients one day that were on insulin for diabetes and I had to prescribe steroids for sudden hearing loss. I made sure to do their complete notes right away. I immediately sent them to the primary care doctors in order for the PCPs to coordinate their diabetes care. In an emergency situation, the patient obviously comes first. However, you need to do your documentation as soon as possible. If I'm urgently taking a patient to surgery from the ED, I might need to know the history obtained from the family member and what meds were already given. I then need to document my procedure so the ICU taking care of the patient post-op knows what has been done and any potential complications to watch for. Some of this communication may be done verbally at first, but it needs to get into the medical record as soon as possible.

What do you actually need to document? You should obviously document everything you did and everything you think is important. We will discuss the things you are required to document for billing/coding purposes a little later. If the patient is verbally abusive or says things that don't make sense, it's great to use quotes. I've put sentences in my notes like, "Patient states, 'You don't know s**t about that. This is a f***ing waste of time.'" Or, "Patient reports, 'I see small bugs coming out of my nose.'" This is a non-judgmental way of accurately documenting a potentially important part of your encounter. It's perfectly appropriate to document if a patient made you feel uncomfortable or if you had to bring an escort into the room. It is not wrong to document that a patient is obese, as that is likely important to their overall health. However, try to state things as objectively as possible. I write, "Strong tobacco odor" in my exam rather than, "Patient reeks of stale cigarettes."

2. Coding overview

Depending on where you work, you may be more or less involved in doing your own coding. Most employers have a coder (or coding department) who will either enter codes themselves or check your codes. Some employers require you to enter a level of service for each outpatient and inpatient encounter, and enter all procedures. This may be done by entering numerical codes, specific keywords/terminology, or choosing the complexity of the interaction. However the codes are entered, you need to make sure your documentation supports whatever code you are choosing. We'll talk about how to do that with as little difficulty as possible.

Coding is done both for patient encounters and procedures. Procedural coding is easier, but still requires some explanation. Encounter coding is called E/M, for Evaluation/Management. This applies to inpatient, outpatient, and emergency room visits. In the end, you are asked how much effort you put into the interaction to come up with an overall "level of service" (LOS). E/M coding can be based on time or "components." If you spend a lot of time with each patient, time-based coding is going to be your best bet. It's relatively easy. For most people, though, you will get a higher level of service if you use components. Unfortunately, component-based E/M coding is an "anti-intuitive" process. Although it eventually asks you how complicated the visit was, the answer to that question is not obvious. It is not, "That one seemed pretty straightforward since it's something I do all the time." The answer comes from adding up a bunch of points. I will teach you how to do that so it requires minimum thought to correctly calculate your score at the end, but it's kind of annoying when you're not very familiar with it. Even if you are not required to calculate the score yourself, you should know how to earn the points in your documentation so the coders can correctly give you credit for what you've done.

Where does all this coding come from? It is from CMS, or Centers for Medicare & Medicaid Services. I have included links to their guidelines in the appendix. The later coding sections will tell you when to refer to them. Although private insurers are not officially bound by CMS guidelines, most follow their lead. Essentially, if you follow the CMS guidelines in your documentation, you will be set for the private insurers, as well.

Disclaimer: In discussing coding with my peers across a variety of specialties, I am fairly knowledgable overall by comparison. However, each specialty has its own particular coding challenges. For example, I know that PCPs do a lot of "well visits." I'll come right out and say that I have no idea how to code those. Make sure you talk to other doctors in your specialty and your local coder to figure out these particular issues.

3. Procedural coding

This applies to procedures done in the operating room, clinics, ER, endoscopy suite, or anywhere else you do something to a patient beyond taking a history and performing an exam. Procedures can be anything as simple as ear piercing (seriously, they used this as an example in one of the new hire general EMR training classes I went through) to as complex as a heart transplant. In your residency/fellowship, you should learn from your attendings in your specialty what actually qualifies as a procedure that needs to be documented, and hopefully how to accurately document it. If you are a surgeon or in another procedure-heavy field, you will likely get familiar with this quickly, as you are usually required to log your cases as you go along.

Each procedure has a unique CPT code. CPT stands for current procedural terminology. These are 5-digit numerical codes, and 2-digit modifiers can be added. These codes officially change each year, but most changes are minor. New codes are sometimes added, and others are deleted or revised. Good EMR systems will allow you to look up codes by either entering the CPT code itself or portions of the words that describe the codes. There is a large book that lists the CPT codes each year. Your employer should have a copy of this available for your use. You can often look up CPT codes with a Google search, but that can be kind of spotty. You are more likely to get the accurate code if you know how to use the CPT book. I use Google when I already know the exact procedure I've done, but don't remember the number (e.g. excision of malignant lesion from lips, 1.5 cm). However, the CPT book is much more complete and informative. It is organized by body system and lists related codes together. There is also a large index that will show you all of the pages in the book where a certain word is located. This helps you choose the code that most accurately reflects what you have done by showing you all of the options available. It also tells you the exclusions, which is helpful. Each code has an RVU value associated with it (actually several different values depending on the setting, but don't worry too much about that). These theoretically reflect the complexity level, but that doesn't actually pan out well in the real world.

One important concept in procedural coding is bundling. When logging your cases as a resident, you are taught to "un-bundle." As a resident, your goal is to log everything you've done. So if I as a resident did a tympanomastoidectomy with ossicular chain reconstruction, I would log 3 codes: tympanoplasty, mastoidectomy, and ossicular chain reconstruction. However, billing 3 codes for this on an actual billing sheet would be fraud. In the real world, many procedures have been bundled together into a single code. Again, this is where the CPT book (or a particularly well-designed surgeon-friendly EMR) comes in handy to see which codes are actually out there. Whether you are choosing the code yourself vs. a coder doing it, your documentation needs to support the code. A coder may contact you if more information is needed.

Exclusions are a similar concept to bundling. You are prohibited from billing for certain procedures at the same time. For example, if you log CPT 30140 for nasal turbinate reduction, you cannot also code CPT 30930 nasal turbinate outfracture. If you do both procedures at the same time, document it in your operative report, but you have to choose which you will actually bill for (generally choosing the higher value code). Why do payors exclude codes? Probably to make it more confusing. Just use the CPT book and it will tell you which ones are excluded. Your coder should know, too. Should...

There is also something known as a global period for procedures. The global period can be from 0 to 90 days depending on the procedure. If a patient is seen in an outpatient or inpatient visit specifically related to the procedure within the global period, you cannot charge the E/M for that visit. A great website call the

Physician Fee Schedule Search (link in index) can tell you the global period for each CPT code, as well as RVU values. Choose "Payment Policy Indicators" for the "Type of Info," and one of the things it lists is global period. The CPT code of interest is entered as the "HCPCS code" on the site. There is also a downloadable help file if you need assistance using the tool.

There are several 2-digit modifiers used in procedural coding. Your surgical coder should be adding these as necessary, but make sure you have the documentation so he or she knows what to do. The first is for bilateral procedures. Certain procedures (e.g. tonsillectomy) are automatically considered bilateral. Other are unilateral by default (e.g. sphenoidotomy). So if you do a bilateral sphenoidotomy, you need to make sure you document that, and the coder will add the bilateral modifier (50) to the 5-digit CPT code. The modifier 51 is used when you perform multiple procedures at the same time. Your surgical coder will generally choose the highest RVU procedure, and then add 51 to any additional codes. There are also codes for using 2 surgeons, "unusual" procedures, and aborting cases. You can look these up in the CPT book if you are interested.

4. E/M Coding

Physicians are often asked to do more of the E/M coding than actual surgical coding. Even if you're not choosing codes yourself, you need to know what the coders are looking for. Specific elements are required for each level of service. Omitting a small piece of information may change your visit from a level 5 to a level 1.

– *New vs. Established*
For E/M codes, the first thing you need to figure out is if a patient is 'new' vs. 'established.' 'New' in this sense means that in the past 3 years, no one in your group has seen this patient, and you personally have not seen this patient when you were part of a different practice in the same specialty. Your 'group' is defined as all physicians working for the same employer in the same specialty

and subspecialty. An established patient has been seen within the past 3 years by you or someone in your group. Some insurers and practices also allow for consult codes, whereby a patient who has been seen in the past 3 years can be billed as a 'consult' instead of 'established' if specific criteria are met (to be discussed later).

Let's look at some examples, since even this first question can be a little tricky.
Example 1: You were employed as a general surgeon at Mercy Hospital and you personally saw patient X in 2017. You then decided to start your own private practice as a general surgeon and see the same patient X in 2018. This would be an established patient since you personally saw him within the past 3 years.
Example 2: You work at Mercy Hospital as a nephrologist. Dr. Takata worked at Mercy Hospital as a nephrologist and retired last year. You see a patient in 2018 that he saw in 2016. Even if you never worked together, this is an established patient since the patient was seen less than 3 years ago by the same specialty in the same department.
Example 3: You are a private practice cardiologist at A1 Cardiology. Dr. Nagi is also a cardiologist, but works at the rival group B2 Cardiology. You see a patient that Dr. Nagi saw last year. This would actually be a NEW patient for you since you and Dr. Nagi work for different groups.
Example 4: You saw patient X on June 1, 2015. You next see patient X again on June 3, 2018. No one in your group has seen patient X between these 2 visits. This has been longer than 3 years, so patient X would be coded as a new patient.
Example 5: You work at the multi-specialty group Super Docs as a urologist. You see patient X. The next week, one of the oncologists also employed by Super Docs sees patient X. Since you are in different specialties, this is a new patient to the oncologist (as long as none of the other oncologists at Super Docs have seen the patient in the past 3 years).

Midlevels and closely-related specialties are tricky for coding new vs. established. For example, NPs are sometimes considered their own 'group.' Therefore, a patient who has seen an NP in one department at a practice might already be considered established if they see an NP who works at a completely different department in the practice. A pulmonologist working in critical care may or may not be the same 'group' as a pulmonologist working at the same hospital's outpatient asthma center. If you have midlevels in your group or work in a potentially overlapping specialty, ask your coders for advice.

Is your head spinning yet? If so, go back to the "Taking care of yourself" section and come back here a little later. A lot of the coding information takes time to process. Practice using it definitely helps, too!

– *Location of Service*
In addition to new vs. established, you have to determine the location of service. The most common locations are outpatient, inpatient, and emergency room. There are different E/M codes for each location, so make sure you are using the right one. Thankfully, this part is usually easier. Keep in mind that even if your clinic is in the hospital, it is an outpatient encounter if the patient is not admitted. The three main locations share similarities in the required documentation, but there are some differences, both in content and time requirements.

– *Time-Based Billing*
Once you've figured out new vs. established and service location, you choose if you are going to bill based on time or components. The documentation side of time billing is far easier than component billing, but time-based billing will usually result in a lower level of service. Also, time-based billing can only be used when over 50% of the visit time was spent in "counseling and/or coordination of care." For outpatients, the total time is only the face-to-face time. For inpatients, all of your 'floor time' counts (i.e. calling consults, charting, rounding or other team discussions on that particular patient). The handy table from AAFP in the appendix lists the required minimum time for each level of service. It is a round down process. As an example, if you spend 18 minutes with a new patient, the correct time-based code would only be 99201 (level 1). As long as you document appropriately, it's usually hard to get less

than a level 3 for a new patient with component-based coding. This is not true with time-based billing.

If you decide time-based billing is the way to go for a particular encounter, your entire documentation could be as brief as the following: "I spent 47 minutes with the patient, 30 of which consisted of counseling regarding the new diagnosis of thyroid cancer." The required elements are, 1) total length of time of encounter in minutes, 2) number of minutes spend in counseling/coordination of care, 3) the specific phrase 'counseling' and/or 'coordination of care' to let readers know this is how you are billing, and 4) what was addressed (i.e. the patient's diagnosis). Technically, the statement in quotes would 'earn' you a level 4 visit if this was a new patient. However, if that is your whole note, you're not really doing things in the spirit of documentation. If this is a new patient, you probably took some sort of history and did an exam. You also might want to know looking back on your note what sort of things you discussed with the patient, such as lab tests, biopsy results, specialist referrals, or prognosis. So your time-based notes should still be informative, but you don't have to worry about checking off a bunch of boxes to figure out your level of service.

Most outpatient physician practices are based on the model of seeing as many patients as possible. Therefore, you won't generally have 45 to 60 minutes with a new patient. I have seen longer visits more commonly in certain specialties (oncology and psychiatry come to mind), so physicians with that type of schedule may tend to use time-based billing more often. Although you must make a choice for each encounter which type of billing you will use (time-based or component-based), you don't have to exclusively use either type for all of your patients. You can even use different types for the same patient on different visits. For example, if you are seeing Ms. Perez for a sick visit, you might use component-based billing. However, if she comes back another time because she has a lot of questions about her new diabetes regimen, you might code that visit using time.

– *The Three Elements*
Unfortunately not as fun as the similarly-named Bruce Willis sci-fi movie, there are 3 elements that are evaluated for E/M coding. They are the past medical history, physical exam, and medical decision making. Each element has its own set of items that determine the overall complexity of that particular section. There are currently two widely-used guideline systems that tell you what you need to document: the CMS 1995 guidelines and 1997 guidelines. The 95 guidelines were felt by some to be too general, so the 97 guidelines are much more specific in what is required, mainly in the exam section. PDF links to both guidelines are in the appendix.

Should you read the guidelines if you never have? Probably. Are they fascinating and full of clarity? Umm... Are they a great source to figure out your code for each visit? Not quite. Once you know the general guidelines of coding (which I will be providing over the next few pages), it is much easier to create a template and then work off a chart to determine your level of service. The guidelines (and charts) use the terms, "problem focused, expanded problem focused, detailed, and comprehensive" for history and exam, and, "straightforward, low complexity, moderate complexity, and high complexity" for medical decision making. These words don't mean what you think they mean, though. They are based on checking off boxes. So my advice is to forget the words and use a chart to figure out what level of service your documentation supports. Although the charts include these words, some also include the actual codes and/or level of service you're using. I have been fortunate to receive some of these charts from my employers, so I keep a copy at my desk. I rarely have to refer to them at this point, but I still use them every now and then when I'm doing something uncommon. I checked with my former employer and learned that their charts are proprietary, so I cannot share them with you here. However, I created my own chart for the MDM section, which I have included in the index. I will explain how to use it later.

– History
The history section includes the following elements: chief complaint, history of present illness (HPI), review of systems, past medical history, social history, and family history. Medical history, surgical

history, medications, and allergies are all included within the past medical history section. Your complexity level in the history section is based on how many of these elements you document in your note.

The HPI is basically what has been happening with the patient that prompted the visit. The chief complaint may be included within the HPI or listed somewhere else in the note. In the real world, the patient is usually "telling her story." In the coding world, the HPI is broken down into 8 elements. These are location, duration, timing, severity, quality, context, modifying factors, and associated signs/symptoms. For level 1 and 2 new patient exams (CPT 99201 and 99202), you must include 1 to 3 of these elements. For levels 3 through 5, you need 4 or more elements. So what are each of these things? Here you go:

Location: site of problem or pain (e.g. right arm)
Duration: how long this has been a problem or when it was noticed (e.g. growth first noticed 2 months ago)
Timing: how it has changed over time (e.g. better, worse, or unchanged since it started)
Severity: can be on a numeric scale (e.g. pain 3/10) or verbal (minor to severe symptom)
Quality: further explanation of symptom – often used with pain (e.g. throbbing, stabbing, burning, or tingling sensation) or unclear/vague symptoms (e.g. "Patient describes dizziness as 'feeling of head fullness and like she is going to fall over.'")
Context: the setting in which symptom occurs (e.g. Patient first noticed back pain when he started driving to more distant work site.)
Modifying factors: things that make the symptom better or worse (e.g. medications, rest, time of day)
Associated signs/symptoms: other things patient has noticed that might be related to main complaint (e.g. in patient with hearing loss, these may include tinnitus, vertigo, ear pain, or ear drainage)

So now that you know what CMS considers important in a history, how do you make sure you've documented it? It's usually pretty easy to get at least 4 of these elements, so the real key is just to document what you have already done. You can either do this in a story fashion and hope that the coder agrees with you, or you can spell it out and make it obvious.

Here is an example of the freeform version that would qualify as a level 5 HPI:
"The patient presents with 3 weeks of worsening left wrist pain not alleviated by ibuprofen."

Wow! This is really short. This shows that documentation does not necessarily have to be lengthy, but it does have to hit certain elements. We have included 4 of the elements above – location (left wrist), duration (3 weeks), timing (worsening), and modifying factors (no help with ibuprofen). We would likely include more information as most patients do not provide us with this concise of a history, and there is often more information we want to know (e.g. any numbness or restricted motion, history of trauma, severity of the pain).

If someone just looked at our HPI above, they would think it was brief. In the CMS coding guidelines, "brief" means that something contains only 1-3 elements. This is an example of the coding guidelines not meaning what you think they mean. Personally, I have made my note templates include at least 4 of the elements so I make sure I hit them and coders have an easy time finding them.

Here is an example of what my HPI might look like:
"Chief complaint: Neck mass. Duration: started 2 months ago. Timing: worse over time - getting larger. Location: right side of neck. Associated symptoms: denies pain at the site."

Since I am usually typing my HPI as the patient is talking to me, my notes usually have more text than the above example. I let them tell me what they feel is important first, and then ask follow up questions if they haven't given me all of the information I want. Generally, for more complex or vague symptoms, you are going to want to type more to get a better understanding. Direct quotes can be helpful when a patient is describing a symptom. For something like a neck mass, though, you might not need a lot of extra text.

The next part of your history is the review of systems (ROS). There are 14 systems recognized by CMS: Constitutional symptoms (e.g., fever, weight loss), Eyes, Ears/Nose/Mouth/Throat, Cardiovascular, Respiratory, Gastrointestinal, Genitourinary, Musculoskeletal, Integumentary (skin and/or breast), Neurological, Psychiatric, Endocrine, Hematologic/Lymphatic, and Allergic/Immunologic. ROS is not required for a level 1 new patient exam. One system must be reviewed for level 2, 2-9 for level 3, and 10 or more for levels 4 and 5. Again, the best way to document this is building it into your template. There are many ways to do this. You can have your patient fill out a ROS form each time they come in, and have your medical assistant input the information. Many EMRs have ROS templates built in, so if you make the patient sheet line up with the computer template, it is very easy to fill in. You can personally go through and ask your patient all of the ROS questions, but this can take a lot of time. For documentation, you can choose to include the entire list of each system, or use a simpler statement like, "A 10-point review of systems was obtained, and is negative except for fever and sore throat." You will probably want to ask some of the problem-related ROS (e.g. if they come in with stomach pain, you would likely ask about diarrhea, vomiting, fever, etc.). You might choose to include this in the HPI section, but to be sure you get "credit" for your ROS, it is safest to specifically mention it as a ROS and how many systems were reviewed.

The final history section includes family history, social history, and "other." The "other" section includes current/prior medical problems, surgical history, current medications, and allergies. For levels 1 and 2 new patients, none of this is required. For level 3, you must include at least 1 component. For levels 4 and 5, you must include 1 element of each of the 3 sections (family, social, and "other"). Many people have their note templates set up so all of this information is pulled in automatically. (Ask your EMR trainer/specialist how to do this if you don't know how. It's slightly different for each EMR system.) You can do this if you want, but I don't like this method. First, it causes very long redundant notes. I don't necessarily want to see every surgery my 90-year-old patient has ever had, as well as every over-the-counter vitamin a patient takes. If this information is already in the chart, I don't need it all in my note. Second, if the chart is not complete, you may think you've hit all of your points only to find that you have not. I have seen many charts where the family history section is blank. So even if you use a link to pull in family history to your note, if no one has entered any family history, you will not be able to code as a level 4 or 5 note.

The way I do this history section makes a lot more sense to me. I look through the chart sections to see if there is anything relevant to the reason I am seeing the patient. If you are a PCP, all of the history may be relevant to you. As a surgical specialist, that's usually not the case. Then I specifically make a comment on smoking status (part of the social history that's usually important to me as an ENT) and relevant family history. So for me, this part of my note template is as follows:

"Past medical history, surgical history, medications, allergies, and social history have been reviewed. History notable for ___. Family history is notable for (history of/no history of) ___."

For the blanks, I have drop down menus that include common items, as well as a free-text field. So for a patient seeing me for hoarseness, the first blank might be filled in with, "current smoker, GERD," and the family history, "no history of head and neck cancer." My whole medical/family social history only takes up 2 lines in my note, and does a good job summarizing the relevant information.

CMS does NOT require you to put the patient's entire history in your note, but you do need to comment that you have reviewed it. I have had coders tell me that you must include something specific, and not just say that you have reviewed it. My method is a very easy way to do that, and I have never had a coder argue with me about it. The same is true with family history. I don't need to document each medical affliction of each of the patient's family members, but I need to include at least 1 piece of information in family history.

– Physical Exam

This is the main difference between the 1995 and 1997 CMS guidelines. Both use terms of "problem-focused," "expanded problem-focused," "detailed," and "comprehensive" to describe the level of physical exam documentation. However, the difference between a "detailed" and "comprehensive" exam was subjective in the 1995 guidelines. The 1995 definitions of detailed and comprehensive exams are as follows:

Detailed – an extended examination of the affected body area(s) and other symptomatic or related organ system(s).
Comprehensive – a general multi-system examination or complete examination of a single organ system.

The 1995 guidelines also list the recognized body areas and organ systems. Basically, the problem with this system was that it was very subjective as to what actually qualified as each level of physical exam. One physician may think his exam is "comprehensive," while the coder may think it is only "detailed." Different coders might disagree with each other, too, as there is no rubric to tell who is right. Also, a "comprehensive" exam from physician X might look totally different from a "comprehensive" exam from physician Y. I initially used the 1995 guidelines for my exam template, but the coders at my institution said that I could not do so. Technically, any individual is legally able to use either 95 or 97 guidelines, but if the coders at your institution aren't familiar with 95, it is going to be a lot less headache for you just to use 97.

The 1997 guidelines made the exam level requirements much clearer as they went to a bullet point system. Basically, the number of bullet points you include determines the level of your exam. They have both a general physical exam and specialty-specific exams. As an ENT, I'm never doing a gastrointestinal or genitourinary exam on my patients, so I always use the ENT-specific template. These templates can be found in the 1997 guidelines link in the index.

To make my exam template that I use for all new patients, I read through the 1997 guideline requirements for the level 4/5 exam. I pasted it into a note and summarized the points. My note then includes the summary, and that I examined all of the listed structures, which were, "normal except as follows ___." Then the only thing I have to type in is anything abnormal. I feel like this makes my notes more readable, and it also makes sure I don't forget anything. I try to do the same exam on all new patients. Obviously if I omit something, I change that in my note. If you want to see how this actually looks, I have included my exam template in the appendix. You can do this for any specialty-specific exam.

Another reasonable option is to build or use a template that has all of the bullet points. Then you can click through each one and say it is normal or what is abnormal in the system. CMS specifically mentions that you can't just say something is "abnormal," but that you must document what the abnormality is. This is the method I usually see from emergency medicine notes, but it is more cumbersome for me personally. It works very well for some people, so feel free to experiment with both systems and see what you like. I do strongly recommend using some sort of template, though, so you don't accidentally omit anything.

One final point on the exam: Sometimes it is impossible to get a part of the exam. If a patient is intubated, I can't do a laryngeal mirror exam on them, as the larynx is blocked by the endotracheal tube. If a pediatric patient has clamped her mouth closed so tightly that the parents and I can't get it open, I can't document a tonsil exam. In these situations, you get credit for the exam you attempted. Make sure not to write 'deferred,' though, as that shows lack of effort rather than impossibility. I would say in my note, "Unable to perform mirror exam due to intubation," or, "Unable to examine oropharynx due to lack of patient cooperation." As long as you document that you tried, you get credit for it. Vital signs are part of the exam, too. Make sure your staff is getting vital signs, or you won't be able to code any higher levels of service.

– Medical Decision Making
This is the more complex part of coding. Guess what – it's divided into 3 parts, you have to add up points, and one of the parts explodes into a ton of bullet points. Are you excited yet? It's OK. You can do it. Also, I made a chart to help you. You may want to refer to it while reading through this section. It's on the last page of the book, or you can print out a separate full-size page using the link on the page right before the chart.

As we discussed above, the history and exam sections can easily be templated into your notes. This cannot really be done with medical decision making (MDM). Some people will have a 'data review' section in their notes, but that does not give you the overall MDM score. I recommend using a sheet and counting up points when you are starting out. Once you do it often enough, you will rarely have to look at the sheet.

MDM 1) Diagnoses and treatment options

Diagnoses are divided into self-limited, established, or new. I was told by coders that self-limited is never really used, or only used for something like a hangnail. Their reasoning was that a reasonable patient would not go to a doctor for something that is truly self-limited. I'm not sure that this is true, but you may want to ask your coder or use your own judgment. The main categories we use are new vs. established. Unlike determining if a PATIENT is new or established, where the patient is new or established to your group, the DIAGNOSIS is new or established to the *individual physician*. Why do they do this? Probably to confuse us. But it is important, because it can drastically change your level of service. We'll show this a little later with examples.

Established problems are worth 1 point each if they are stable or improved, and 2 points each if they are worsening. New problems are worth 3 points each if no additional workup is planned, and 4 points each if additional workup is planned. Each diagnosis you address at the visit is categorized into 1 of these 4 categories (5 if you include the "self-limited" category), and you add up all the points. So for any given visit, you can go from 1 to very, very many points (if your patient has a lot of diagnoses). The rubric only cares whether you get 1, 2, 3, or 4+ points, so you can stop adding once you reach 4. Make sure you remember to document each diagnosis for the encounter in order to get credit.

Let's show some examples for adding up points in this MDM section.
1. My partner (same private practice, same specialty) saw patient X for epistaxis 2 weeks ago. The patient follows up with me today for

epistaxis, but this is the first time I am seeing this patient. The patient reports she is getting better, and nothing further needs to be done. The patient will be an established patient, but epistaxis will be a NEW diagnosis in MDM since I have not seen this patient for this problem. So for me to see this patient, I get 3 points in MDM part 1. My partner would only get 1 point.

2. Dr. Sheir is a PCP seeing her patient Dolores. Dolores is coming in for a new shoulder pain issue, but also has diabetes. Dr. Sheir chooses to get an X-ray for the shoulder pain, and also documents Dolores' stable recent blood sugar checks. The points would be 4 for the new shoulder pain with additional workup and 1 for the established stable diabetes. This is 5 points total. In counting, Dr. Sheir can just stop at the shoulder pain since she already had 4 points, but she obviously wants to document for clinical purposes the fact that she addressed the chronic problem.

3. Special case: escalation of care. Dr. Chan has seen patient Arnold for hypertension twice. They tried diet and exercise, but Arnold's blood pressure is still not under control. Dr. Chan decides that Arnold needs to be started on an antihypertensive. It could be argued that this is only 1 point (established problem, stable), but coders have told me that the 1 point "stable" is really more like "happily stable." Arnold's blood pressure hasn't really gotten worse in this scenario, but it is not getting better, so you are having to escalate care. Coders have told me that this would actually get 2 points, since "established, worsening" also involves escalation of care.

MDM 2) Amount and/or Complexity of Data to Be Reviewed

This is the second point system within MDM. Basically, you get points for the data and information you obtain and review outside of taking the history directly from the patient – only if you document it, of course. I'll explain how the points work and how you add them up properly.

Reviewing or ordering lab tests (bloodwork, pathology): 1 point

Reviewing or ordering imaging tests (X-ray, CT, MRI, PET, etc): 1 point
Reviewing or ordering "medicine" tests (EKG, EEG, audiogram – essentially any test that's not tissue/blood or radiology): 1 point
Even if you review all of the blood work your patient has ever had done and you order 5 new lab tests, that is only 1 point for this section. You'll probably get more points somewhere else, but you can only get 1 point for each of these types of tests. However, if you order an X-ray, review a CBC, and review an EKG, that's 3 points total since they're each in separate sections.

If you independently visualize/interpret an image or study yourself, you actually get 2 points for that. For example, let's say my patient had a CT scan of his neck. I look at the images myself, and I also look at the CT report generated by the radiologist. As long as I document my interpretation (which could be something as simple as "no neck mass seen"), I get 3 points for this – 2 for my independent visualization of the image and 1 for the review of the radiology test. This is what I usually write in my note:
"CT neck from [date] was personally reviewed by me. My interpretation shows no suspicious neck masses. Report also reviewed – as above."

This comes up commonly for radiology, but is also true for other studies. If you interpret the EKG yourself rather than just looking at the report, you can get credit for that. As an ENT, I commonly do this for audiograms in addition to imaging studies. Sleep studies, EEGs, ABIs, and any other test where there is raw data available are all candidates.

The final group in this point system relates to your information sources. Here are the points:

Discussion of test results with performing physician: 1 point
Discussion of case with another health care provider: 2 points
Decision to obtain records/history from someone other than the patient: 1 point
Obtaining history from someone other than the patient: 2 points
Summary of old records: 2 points

If you call the pathologist to discuss the results, you get 1 point (in addition to your 1 point above for review of pathology). If you call the patient's PCP to discuss the case rather than just sending your office note, you get 2 points. If you document that you *decide* to get information from a source other than the patient, it is worth 1 point. (This one seems kind of strange. The only time I really use it is when I say that part of the plan is to get records from somewhere.) If you actually *get* information from another person or look at and summarize old records, you get 2 points. The "other person" could be a parent for a pediatric patient, a spouse, or anyone else who comes to the office visit if they are providing a significant amount of history. Interpreters also count in this category.

The two points for record summary/review are separate from review of lab/imaging data, but you must state what you reviewed. If a PCP refers a patient to you and you review the PCP's note, documentation of that review earns you 2 points. The key is that you have to summarize what you reviewed. This does not have to be long, but it can't just be, "Reviewed PCP's note." An acceptable format is, "Reviewed PCP's note from [date] – stated normal tonsil exam." If you also reviewed the strep test – and documented it – that's another point.

Strangely enough, review/summary of records, obtaining history from someone other than the patient, and discussion of case with another provider are all listed together. So even if you do all 3 of these things, you only get 2 points total for that work. Once you have done your documentation, add up the points. Like in the first MDM category, only points 1-4 matter. Once you get to 4, you can stop counting. Time for a couple examples.

1. A Russian-speaking patient comes to see you. An interpreter is used for the visit. The patient's spouse tells you all of the medications the patient takes. You also look at the PCP's referral note. Points: 2. This is because obtaining the history from the interpreter and the spouse as well as summarizing old records are all included in the same 2-point category.
2. A patient brings records from their prior doctor. You look through them and see a cardiology office visit, coagulation studies, and an

echocardiogram report. You document, "Reviewed old records - Cardiology visit last year reported patient cleared for outpatient surgery. Coags and echo normal." Although abbreviations are not great, it is actually worth 4 points – 2 for review of summary of old records, 1 for review of labs, 1 for review of "medicine" test.

3. You see a 5-year old for a sore throat. His dad provides the history. You order a rapid strep test. You also look through the chart and see the patient has had 3 positive strep tests in the past year. Your documentation includes, "Father provides history," "Strep test ordered," and "3 positive strep tests in past year." Points: 3 total; 2 for obtaining history from someone other than the patient, and 1 for ordering/reviewing labs. You can only get 1 point per visit for labs, no matter how many you order or review.

MDM 3) Risk of Complications and/or Morbidity or Mortality ("Risk")

The final component of medical decision making is basically the seriousness/danger of the diagnosis or treatment. This is a large table published by CMS (page 47 in the 97 guidelines). It includes the risk/severity of three areas: presenting problem(s), diagnostic procedure(s) ordered, and management option(s) selected. At least you don't have to add any points for this category. The highest level of risk in any of the categories determines the overall risk for this section of MDM. The confusion in this area is correlating a point value or qualitative risk level with your overall visit code. Keeping that in mind, I will designate 4 as the highest risk level here, since 4 is the highest number of points you ever need to worry about in the other MDM sections. I included all the entries from the CMS table in my MDM table, so you can use the single MDM table both to find the risk level and to calculate your overall MDM score.

The easiest way to use this table is to know where the interventions you commonly use fall in the risk ranking. This will be different for you depending on your specialty and type of practice. For me as an ENT, things I commonly do include over-the-counter medications, prescription medication management, referral for physical therapy, office endoscopy, and both minor and major surgery. Also, I conveniently put the highest risk level on the top line. Since only the highest value matters for the risk component of MDM, just read across the Risk section and stop as soon as you get to something you documented doing in that visit.

Most of the entries in the table are fairly straightforward, but I will clarify a few for you based on what I've learned from coders over the years.

– Prescription drug management: The most obvious example is prescribing a medication. However, telling someone to stop or continue a prescription also counts, whether it was prescribed by you or someone else.
– Minor vs. major surgery: I was told by some coders that major surgery can be considered anything that requires general anesthesia. However, another coder told me that ear tubes in a child were not major surgery even though we need to use a general anesthetic. A surgery can still be major surgery if it is done with local or regional anesthesia. So the best thing to do here is use your judgement and ask your coders.
– "Identified risk factors" for endoscopy or surgery: These are things that make the procedure more dangerous. This often relates to patient co-morbidities, such as obesity, poor cardiac status, genetic syndromes, or anticoagulant use. If you feel like your patient has a risk factor, you should document it to support your coding choice. For example, "Discussed higher risk of poor wound healing in cosmetic surgery due to patient's tobacco use."

Examples determining the Risk component:

1) Dr. Haskins is an ophthalmologist who sees a patient with glaucoma. He performs tonometry in the office to check the eye pressure, which is stable. He tells the patient to continue his current prescription eye drop. This would be level 3 risk due to the prescription drug management. The single chronic problem and tonometry are lower risk than the prescription management, so they do not figure into the calculation.

2) Janet presents to the emergency room with severe flank pain. She is diagnosed with a kidney stone using an ultrasound. The ED

doctor gives her a dose of IV morphine for the pain. This is level 4 risk due to the use of a parenteral controlled substance. Again, the low-risk diagnosis of kidney stone and minimal-risk diagnostic test of ultrasound do not matter since the IV morphine is in a higher-risk category.

3) Paul was playing soccer in his high school gym class. He got hit with a ball in the head and briefly lost consciousness. He has a normal neurologic exam and only a minor bruise on his forehead. His pediatrician and mother discuss CT scan, but decide just to observe at home. This is level 3 risk due to the loss of consciousness, even though no testing or treatment were done.

MDM: Putting it all together

Now you should have two independent point scores and a risk level. We will call these your 3 contributors. How do we determine the overall MDM score? The correct score is the highest level supported by at least 2 out of your 3 contributors. Unfortunately, the way CMS has defined the points is not numerically aligned with the MDM E/M LOS (medical decision making evaluation & management level of service). Here is the break down for that:

Score 1 = E/M level 2
Score 2 = E/M level 3
Score 3 = E/M level 4
Score 4+ = E/M level 5

I am very sorry if you are angry right now at how needlessly complex this is. The good news it that it's not that hard once you get used to it, and it's exactly the same for new patients and established patients. The numbers and table are slightly different when coding for a new hospital admission, but they use the same general idea.

By far the easiest way to do this when you are starting is to have the chart in front of you as you code your encounters. Add up your points in each section, making sure that you have documented in accordance with the points you are giving yourself. Next, find the highest risk level in the risk chart. Then see where the results fall.

If you have 1 point (level 2), 3 points (level 4), and risk level 4, your overall MDM E/M is level 4.
If you have 4 points (level 5), 4 points (level 5), and risk level 1, your overall MDM E/M is level 5.
If you have 2 points (level 3), 0 points (level 1), and risk level 4, your overall MDM E/M is level 3. In this situation, level 3 is the highest level supported by at least 2 of the contributors, so that is the correct level to choose.

– The Three Elements Coding: Putting it all Together
Remember when we discussed that there are 3 elements to determining your overall visit E/M code? Now we have to put them all together. These are the History, Exam, and Medical Decision Making.

Figuring out the MDM E/M level was a prelude to figuring out your overall E/M code. For NEW patients, the correct overall E/M level is the highest level supported by ALL 3 of your elements. As we discussed in the history and exam sections, it is very easy to template in the level 5 history and exam. As long as you hit all of the required sections, the only thing you really need to figure out is your MDM coding. If you have your regular level 5 history and exam for your new patient but your MDM comes out to level 3, the correct code is 99203 (level 3 new patient visit).

There are multiple reasons why I recommend doing it this way. First, when you are seeing a new patient, it is really your duty to be thorough to make sure you are serving them well as a physician. I don't necessarily need to know someone's entire medical or life history as a specialist, but I should learn about why the patient is coming to see me (HPI), relevant PMH/medications, and if there may be some genetic basis/risk to their disease (family history). Smoking status is very relevant to what I do, whether as a risk for head and neck cancer, voice/throat issues, worsening of sinonasal complaints, or healing from surgery. That essentially gives me a level 5 history. Also, I think each new patient deserves a thorough exam. I have found asymptomatic tumors in patients unrelated to their chief complaints just by doing a thorough head & neck exam.

Another reason to do a thorough history and exam for a new patient is to make your documentation and coding easier. If you do the same thing every time, less typing is involved since you already have your template in the note. You only have to change abnormalities. If you don't have to worry about where your history and exam fall, you only have to look at MDM for overall code determination.

Additionally, this is the best way to capture the complexity and time investiture of what you do. If you look at the CMS documents, they use these words like "straightforward," "brief," "comprehensive," "complex." We would all agree that certain patients and scenarios are high risk. If a patient comes in with an acute stroke, she has a high-risk situation that requires rapid, high-quality medical care to achieve the best possible outcome. In my specialty, someone with a new diagnosis of head and neck cancer would generally be considered complex or high risk. In MDM, they have a serious disease, they are likely to have at least a diagnostic surgery/biopsy even if they don't require a major cancer resection, and there will likely be a lot of testing (labs, CT scan, preoperative EKG). Complex planning goes into caring for this patient. If you do a cursory history or exam, you will not be able to code at a high level to compensate you for the time and mental effort required to care for this patient.

On the other hand, seeing a patient with recurrent strep throat and deciding to perform a tonsillectomy might be considered a "straightforward" situation for an ENT if you think about it in the regular way we use the word "straightforward." However, a lot actually goes into this encounter. You can usually make this decision the first time you see a patient if you have documentation of an adequate history of infections. You'll get 3 points for this being a new problem without additional workup, and your intervention of major surgery (without risk factors) is level 3 risk. As long as you take a good history and do a good exam, you are going to get a level 4 visit (99204) from the above documentation. This is part of why it's useful to go through the points and table rather than just using CMS's arbitrary descriptions.

So for me, new patient coding is very easy. I always do a level 5 history and exam, and then I just have to figure out my MDM level. Whatever the MDM level is, that's the overall E/M code level. If you don't want to do it this way, just figure out the level for each section (history, exam, MDM) and then take the highest number supported by each. For example:
History 5, Exam 5, MDM 4: 99204 (wRVU 2.43)
History 5, Exam 2, MDM 4: 99202 (wRVU 0.93)
History 3, Exam 3, MDM 3: 99203 (wRVU 1.42)
Kim's coding – History always 5, Exam always 5, MDM varies per encounter: overall code = code supported by MDM level

I mentioned RVUs (relative value units) earlier as a way that many physicians are paid. There are different types of RVUs (i.e. facility vs. work), but the ones you usually care about as a physician are the wRVUs (work relative value units). Just as a quick demonstration, let's say you see 40 new patients a week, working 40 weeks per year (yes, this sounds like a nice amount of time off). Let's say your average documentation is line 2 above – comprehensive history, limited exam, and "moderate" MDM. In this case, you would earn 1488 RVU for these patients. Let's say you get $60 per wRVU (I have seen numbers both higher and lower than this). This is a total of $89,280 for these patients. Let's say you do line 1 above instead – comprehensive history, comprehensive exam, and "moderate" MDM. These patients now earn you $233,280! That's a huge difference in your salary, just by changing your exam template.

Why do I put this out there? Am I encouraging you to "overcode?" No! It's to get compensated for what you're probably doing already. And technically, undercoding is just as fraudulent as overcoding. What I'm trying to do is make coding more efficient and more rewarding for you.

Now that you're an expert in new patient coding, I'll tell you the main difference with established patient coding. For established patients, the overall level of service is determined by using the highest code supported by only 2 out of the 3 elements (instead of all 3 like in new patients). However, one of these 2 must always be MDM. So what I do for established patients is keep the history the same, so I know that's level 5. I usually do a limited exam (just focusing on the area of interest), and I don't use that in my established patient coding. If the patient is following up for otitis externa, I've already done my complete head and neck exam at their initial visit. I probably only need to look in the ears at this point. This saves time and makes logical sense if everything else was normal at the initial visit. Doing it this way, I still only have to look at MDM to determine my overall E/M code.

If you don't want to do it my way, here are examples for determining the established patient E/M visit code (99211-99215):
History 5, Exam 1, MDM 4: 99214 (use history and MDM)
History 3, Exam 3, MDM 4: 99213 (use MDM and either history or exam)
History 5, Exam 5, MDM 2: 99212 (even though history and exam are 5, you MUST use MDM as one of your 2 elements, so overall level is 2)
Kim's coding – History always 5, Exam score doesn't matter since not using, MDM determined individually at each encounter: overall code = code supported by MDM level

This is a pretty good introduction to outpatient coding. As I mentioned, there are some small differences for other coding scenarios, like inpatient and emergency room. I also have no idea how things like OB visits or "well-child checks" are coded. Make sure to ask your colleagues about these if needed. Documentation requirements are quite similar across all of these arenas, but the actual codes used will differ.

– *Special Situation: Consults*

One other area we can cover relatively briefly is consult codes. Consult coding format is quite similar to new patient coding format, but a few additional criteria apply. First, the patient must have a primary insurance that accepts consult codes. Medicare does not allow use of consult codes, but some private insurers do. Ask the billers at your hospital which of your insurers allow consults if you want to know. Why does it matter? Consult codes have a higher RVU value than new patient codes, which in turn are higher than established patient codes. If you are seeing a lot of patients that can be billed as consults, it is significant financially. It might be the difference of almost $100 for a single patient encounter (billing 99214 (wRVU 1.5) vs. 99244 (wRVU 3.02)). This can really add up.

So what is required for a visit to be a consult? First, the consult must be requested by another provider. The consultant (you) must provide your opinion on the case. You must render your findings/recommendations back to the referring provider. You must NOT take over care of the patient for the issue in question. Let's look at these factors using examples.

Example 1: A patient goes to the emergency room for a broken finger. The emergency room splints the finger, then refers the patient to an orthopedic surgeon for outpatient care. The orthopedic surgeon CANNOT bill this as a consult, because he will NOT be sending the patient back to the emergency room doctor.

Example 2: A patient goes to the emergency room for a broken finger. The emergency room splints the finger, then tells the patient to follow up with his PCP. The PCP sees the patient, then refers the patient to the orthopedic surgeon. The orthopedic surgeon determines that no additional care is needed, and the patient should just follow up with his PCP. As long as the surgeon sends his note back to the PCP and the patient has an insurance that allows consults, this CAN be billed as a consult. This is because the specialist opinion was sought, the specialist did not take over care of the patient, and the specialist sent his recommendations back to the referring physician, who will continue to care for the patient.

Example 3: A patient goes to the emergency room for a broken finger. The emergency room splints the finger, then tells the patient to follow up with his PCP. The PCP sees the patient, then refers the patient to the orthopedic surgeon. The orthopedic surgeon determines that he needs to do surgery for the patient. This CANNOT be billed as a consult, because the specialist has taken over the care of the patient.

An interesting thing about consults is that they can be billed for established patients. Let's say that Dr. Cather, an endocrinologist, saw Miss Shimerda 2 years ago for hypothyroidism. She placed the patient on a low dose of Synthroid, and told the patient to follow up with her PCP, Dr. Burden. Dr. Burden has been caring for Miss Shimerda, but wants her to see endocrinology again because her TSH has been creeping up. Dr. Burden refers the patient back to Dr. Cather. Dr. Cather sees Miss Shimerda and recommends increasing the Synthroid slightly. Dr. Cather sends her note back to Dr. Burden, and Dr. Burden continues to manage the patient. Even though Dr. Cather saw the patient less than 3 years ago, she can bill as a consult code in the above scenario as long as the patient's insurance accepts consults. This is the situation mentioned above where the code might be 99244 (level 4 consult) rather than 99214 (level 4 established patient).

Final coding tip

There is one important modifier you should know if you do any procedures in clinic. If you bill for E/M and a procedure at any visit, you should add the 25 modifier to you E/M code. This shows that you did a "separate, distinct procedure" along with your E/M code. You will likely need to enter to code for the procedure, as well, but it is possible that you will only be paid for the E/M or the procedure if you do not add 25 to the E/M.

SECTION FOUR: Financial (and Life) Planning

You've learned a lot about patient care through your formal medical training, and now you know a lot about how to choose your path, get a job, and do the job, just from reading this book. However, you probably don't want to do the job forever. Also, you want to be happy in the job you're doing. That's what this last section is for – learning to plan your life and finances so you can enjoy your life and not worry about money.

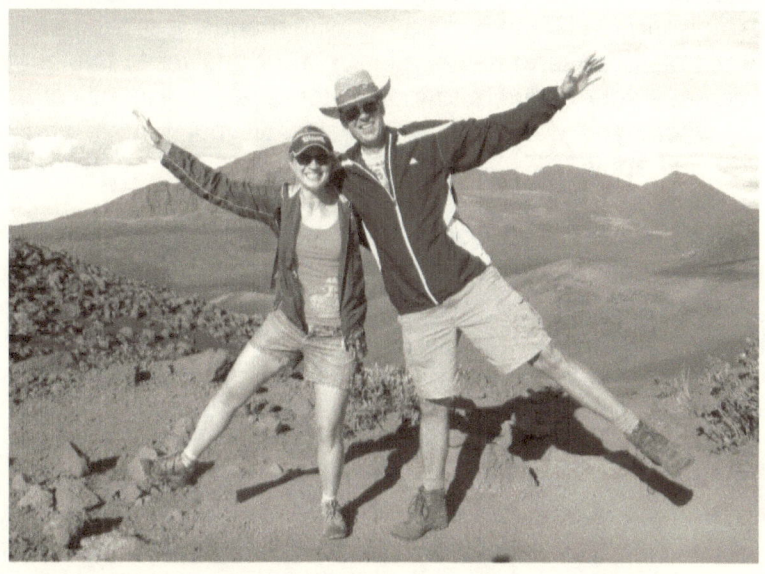

Fun at Haleakala – partially attributable to financial planning!

Chapter One: Life Planning

Sometimes life just happens, but it generally happens more the way you want it to if you do some planning. I've broken this down into some "big picture" questions. You may not have all the answers to these questions right now, and your answers might change over time. It's helpful to start thinking about them early on so you can live the best life possible.

– Who do you want to live with?
Some people really enjoy being on their own. Others want to have a spouse or partner. Some people live with friends or extended family. Many people choose to have children. Your answer to this question will influence your answers to many others, as your family structure affects where you want to live, the size of your house, and what makes you happy.

If you want to have a spouse or partner, this takes work. You might be lucky enough to meet someone during school, but it tends to get progressively harder after that. When you are in residency, it is very challenging to have a social life. You need to be honest and realistic with anyone you are dating about time constraints and lack of freedom in your schedule. Many marriages fail during residency and practice because people do not make them a priority. Medicine is a field where it is easy to be overwhelmed by your schedule and duties, and this is sometimes at the expense of other people in your life. Make sure you are open with your partner and you address issues before they become irreparable. If you have more of a dominating personality (as is true with many of us surgeons, as well as many other physicians) and your partner is more passive, make sure they can still talk to you. You don't want to be shocked by your wife "suddenly" leaving. I married my husband just prior to starting medical school. Residency was really hard, but he was very supportive. We definitely enjoy each other a lot more now, though, since I have finished residency and focused more on doing my career in a way that makes me happy.

Children are probably even more work than a spouse. My husband and I don't have children (by design), so I can only look at others for this. My sister has 3 kids, each 2 years apart. She stays home with the kids, but I still don't know how she does it. One of my good friends from ENT residency had a child during residency, and had a second soon after that. She got 6 weeks of maternity leave during residency, and then was right back at it. She now works full time as a pediatric ENT. He husband is a radiologist. They live in the same city as her in-laws, and they have a nanny during the day. At least with a physician salary you shouldn't have to worry too much about the cost of childcare, but you are still in charge of your children. You need to make sure you are raising them to be happy, responsible people. Hopefully you have people to help you with this during the day – family, friends, or professionals – but I also hope that you want to be part of that process since you chose to have children in the first place. Children will take a huge amount of time, energy, and money, so make sure you are willing to dedicate that to them if you choose to have them.

So if you want to have kids, when should you do it? I have often thought that if you're going to have kids, you should do it while you're young so 1) you have enough energy for it, and 2) you haven't thought or talked yourself out of it! However, medical school and residency are times where you don't have much say in your own schedule. If you choose to have children during these times – especially if you are a woman – you need to make sure you have a plan in place for how your child is going to be cared for day-to-day. As long as you work hard and are resourceful, I truly believe you can do anything you want to do. So don't make what you think is a bad decision, but don't let excuses change your plans for your life. You can always think of a reason why 'now' is not a good time to have a child, but if you keep looking at it that way, you might miss out on your biologic window. Adoption is still an option, but energy levels usually drop with aging, too!

– *Where do you want to live?*
You may have a very specific location in mind. This might be near your extended family, especially if you have children. It may be a specific region of the country you love (like me, in the western US). Maybe you're a big city person, or you prefer a small town. If you're an academic, you might be drawn to a certain program or university.

If you already know your destination city, you just have to find a job there (see Section One). If you don't know where that is, many resources are available to help you find out. The first is obvious – talk to people! You probably have friends, family members, and colleagues scattered throughout the country or the world. Talk to them and see what they like and dislike about where they live. Think about how the person you're speaking to is similar to or dissimilar from you, and apply their information accordingly. Use people you know for informal networking, too. If you hear about an area and want to know more about it, ask your contacts if they know anyone there. This is insanely easy now with social media.

Even if you don't know anyone in a certain place, cities are really easy to research. Wikipedia has an article that lists the 300 largest cities in the US in population order, ranging from 8.4 million in New York City down to 100,000 in Vacaville, CA (see index). You can click on links to each city to learn more about them, and go from there. There are also paper maps (yes, they still exist) that can show you a given area and what all is there. I really like the 50 state road atlases, because I feel like they give you a much better sense of the relative sizes of cities/towns and show you parks and other attractions. Google maps and other map apps are great at getting you from one point to another, but they're not designed for exploring. If you want to investigate specific cities, http://www.city-data.com/ is a great site. You can type in a city name, look on a map of any state, or sort by city size. It has information on weather, crime, employment, demographics, cost of living, and much more.

Once you have narrowed down your search geographically by doing your networking and research, go visit these places. Sometimes you will be pleasantly surprised by a place. On the other hand, you might hate a place you thought you would love. It's less painful to learn this on a visit than after you've packed up a moving van. Talk to people who live there, and ask what they like and dislike about it. If you have learned anything about the city that concerns you (e.g. poor weather, high crime rate), ask people about it. The weather may not be as bad as it sounds, and crime might be focused in one main area of the city.

– What activities are important to you?
Again, this is different for each person. Some people really enjoy restaurants, shows, and sporting events, whereas others want access to nature. I can tell you right now that my small town in southern Oregon does not have a lot of fancy stores. That's fine with me, though. When I was looking to move here, that was something that people repeatedly 'warned' me about. I couldn't care less, but other people have different opinions. If you love boating, you probably shouldn't move to Albuquerque – not much water there. Just make sure you think about what you like to do (or might like to do) and make sure the place you're going has that available.

Travel can be an issue, too. The city where I live has an airport, but it has only intermittent commercial service. We have to drive 90 minutes through a mountain pass to get to the nearest airport. It's small, though, so only offers direct service to about 6 cities. I really like to travel, so this is one of the things I don't like about my town. However, I make it work since I like a lot of other things about this area. If you are working full time as a physician, travel convenience might not be a big deal. However, if your spouse travels for work or you like to fly frequently to visit friends or family, it would probably be more convenient to live closer to a major airport.

Religion is very important to many people. Thankfully, even small towns usually have a wide variety of religious institutions. city-data.com does have faith-specific information on cities, and there are probably other websites with this information. You could ask your local religious leader, as well.

In addition to ensuring that your desired activities are available where you live, you have to make sure you are making time to pursue these activities. This has to do with the work-life balance we discussed in the beginning of Section Three. I think there are very few people who will say that their job is the only activity that is important to them. I know I'm not one of them! Work is indeed important, but there are a lot of other things I enjoy.

– How will you maintain your health?
Again, we discussed caring for yourself earlier in the text. If you need a reminder, go back up to the beginning of Section Three. I just wanted to note a couple things. As with most things in life, good habits start early. However, it's rarely too late to change in this arena. If health is important to you – which I would say it is for most people – you need to work to maintain and potentially improve it. Make sure you are active either at work or outside of it. My husband walks to and from work every day, and I try to work out at least 3 times per week. Make sure you eat well, too. This includes healthful food and reasonable portions. I don't always eat the healthiest items, but by cooking myself, I control how much salt and fat goes into my food. Eating at home also helps with portion control, as you decide how much food goes onto your plate. It's pretty easy to put any leftovers into the fridge, too. If you already have any health problems, most of them don't improve with age. Make sure you are following your doctor's recommendations (since we doctors make such great patients...) and taking steps to reduce your risks of future medical problems. You can talk to your doctor about preventive medicine (which is often covered at low or no-cost with many insurance plans), or do your own research. Finally, you want to consider access to medical care in your community. Some people don't want to live in small towns – especially as they age – as they may have to travel long distances for specialty care.

– How will you react to outside influences?
As adults, we know we cannot control others. We sure wish we could, whether they are our patients or our families. However, this is not going to happen. (Except with kids when they do as they're told and a sufficient reason is, "Because I'm your mom and I said so." I know parents wished this worked all the time!) In interacting with other adults, though, the only thing we can control is how we react to them. If you need help with this, there are many books that provide instructions in constructively reacting to other people. Therapists and other related professionals can help, as well.

There are often bad situations that happen to people, too. I'm often amazed how well some patients handle a cancer diagnosis, whereas others totally freak out if they have to wait 24 hours for an antibiotic to start working for their minor skin infection. Some people lose their job and slide into depression, whereas others get right out there and start searching. Each person has a different baseline resiliency. If you can work on this, you will probably be walking around with a much lower stress level. And when bad things happen, they won't throw you for such a loop. If you are not very good at this now, I can personally recommend this as something to work to improve!

A specific outside influence that happens frequently to physicians is being sued. You have some control over this in treating your patients with respect and honesty in the first place and practicing high-quality medicine, but you cannot stop a patient from suing you. According to a 2018 AMA article (link in appendix), 1/3 of all physicians have been sued. Among surgeons and OB/GYNs, the number is closer to 2/3. The article states that the defendant (the physician) wins in 88% of the cases, but it is still a very stressful situation for a physician. It is also very costly for the system (as most of the costs are handled by malpractice insurance rather than the physician personally), and lawsuits take a lot of time. Being sued usually makes someone worry at first. There's also a sense of betrayal that a patient that you did your best to help turned around and sued you. Then there's the fact that most of what happens during the whole process of the case is out of your hands, and you can't do much to speed it along. If you get sued, take time to process it, but try not to dwell on it. It's like when you have a complication with a patient or any other bad event in your life. You need to acknowledge that it happened, process your feelings, do whatever you can to make it better, accept the things that you cannot change about it, and continue with your life. Sometimes this whole process takes a couple minutes, and other times it can take years.

Again, make sure you get help if you need it. The one caveat with lawsuits is that you want to make sure you don't talk to anyone other than your spouse or legal team about the suit, as they could be deposed if you talk to them. If you are talking to your own physician or therapist about your feelings related to the suit, this should be protected under the physician-patient relationship. It's probably safest to ask your legal team who you should talk to if you need help working through it. However, asking another colleague what they would have done in the situation or telling them about what happened is NOT protected. This is quite annoying, as part of the way we learn as physicians is by talking to other physicians. It's very natural to want to talk to someone who would understand the medical aspects of the case, but you want to avoid this.

– What makes you happy?
Um, probably not getting sued. Let's get off that topic and onto a better one. I'll tell you right now that I was very unhappy during residency. Since you don't have much freedom or free time in residency, I'm not sure how much you can plan for happiness during that time. You can definitely plan for *future* happiness and be ready to implement your plan as soon as possible.

Some people are really lucky and happiness just happens. They are naturally positive people, they have plenty of money, the people in their life are very supportive, and they have minimal health problems. However, we all know people that *should* be happy by all outward appearances, yet are miserable. They have money, friends, health, and success, yet they complain all the time or suffer from depression. Why is this? I think there are two main answers to this question: 1) Different things make different people happy, and 2) Each person has his or her own way of looking at the world.

So to be happy, one part is figuring out what makes you happy. It is much safer and healthier to base your happiness on internal factors, as external factors – health, wealth, other people – can be taken away. Some of these internal or self-directed factors may be taking pride in your work, volunteering in your community, or meditation. Hopefully you enjoy activities with others, as well – hiking with your spouse, attending your child's extracurricular activities, or having friends over for dinner and games – but you want to make sure that at least some of your happiness is based on the way you feel about yourself and your own actions. No one can take those things away from you. Many people think that money makes them happy, but I will say from experience that that is rarely true. I think that it's easier for people to be happy when they don't have to *worry* about money, but the money itself does not buy happiness – just lack of worry about finances. I was making lots of money at my first job out of residency, but I wasn't happy. I'm much happier now making less money and having a better work-life balance under working conditions more of my own choosing.

Some people *think* they know what makes them happy, but they've never actually analyzed those thoughts. You might be tempted to respond with the typical health, wealth, and good relationships. These things make a lot of people happy, but not everyone. Being around horses might make you really happy. Exploring new places might be your thing. Making time to sit quietly and meditate may be someone else's answer. If you've never truly though about it, I encourage you to do so. (And remember, I was the one who said that "mindfulness meditation" just felt like a huge waste of time to me. This is not "touchy-feely-connect-with-your-inner-yogi" advice, this is "figure-out-how-to-be-happy" advice! It's very different.)

If you're not a positive person at baseline, try to become more positive. I guarantee that it will make your life better. We have research that shows that people with a positive attitude have better health outcomes. A Harvard study (see index for link) that followed 70,000 women showed a significantly lower mortality from multiple causes in individuals who were more optimistic. We've probably all heard the saying, "Learn to appreciate the little things (or simple pleasures)." Just the other day, I enjoyed seeing the fall colors, reading a little note my husband wrote me in the morning, and descriptive lines in a book I was reading. You don't have to get a promotion or get engaged to be happy. Also, positive people tend to like being around other positive people. So if you yourself are more positive, you will attract more positive people into your life, and the happiness will multiply.

A fun note on what makes me happy (since I'm writing the book, after all): Last year, I was fortunate to accomplish one of my long-term dreams. One of my first dreams was driving the Oscar Meyer Weinermobile. When I learned how hot dogs were made and subsequently stopped eating them many years ago, I came to the conclusion that driving the Weinermobile might not be a great choice. Somewhere along the years, my dream turned to being a mascot. A couple years ago, I saw that the local college in town was recruiting for people to join the mascot team. I had to wait over 2 long years, but I finally got to be the mascot for the town's winter parade! This was very, very exciting for me. I have since done it several more times for sporting events and another parade. I know it's a strange hobby for a surgeon, but who cares?

– What's your back-up plan?
A side gig as a mascot won't pay the bills, so we should be realistic in addition to being positive. Sometimes our initial plans don't work out. It's always good to have a back-up plan. This can be within your own specialty, within the medical field, or in a totally different area.

I thought that I would be at my first job out of residency for many years. This was not the case. I ended up not being happy there. Some of it was frustration with the contract. From reading this book, you should now know a lot more about contracts than I did when I signed that first one. Hopefully this will help you avoid some of the mistakes I made. Others issues were with some of my coworkers and administrators. I wrote about some of those mistakes in my *Communication in Medicine* book, but I'm not sure how much I could have changed in that situation. Regardless, it's fairly uncommon nowadays that physicians spend a long time at their first job out of residency.

If you are thrilled with your practice, that's great. If not, I encourage you to do two things simultaneously: see what you can improve at your current practice, and look for other options. You don't necessarily want to "give up" on something that can be fixed, but you don't want to be stuck in a bad situation, either. I think I waited too long to start really looking for other jobs once I started disliking my first job. I hoped that I could work things out with my first employer, so didn't seriously look around until I knew I was going to quit. I ended up not working for about 6 months. This was fine since I had money saved, but it might be hard for some people. None of my subsequent employers have mentioned any problem with my 6-month gap, but I always have to explain it on new applications. You want to be careful if it gets to more than 1 year, and especially 2 years, as it can be harder to get licensed or credentialed if you are off for that long.

Options within your specialty may be the same type of job at a different location, or could be something else. Moving from full time to part-time can help, especially if you're feeling symptoms of burnout. On the other hand, you could consider starting your own practice. I have not done this myself, so can't tell you much about it. It's definitely a lot more work, but you do get more freedom. You could also consider clinical versus research positions. There aren't many strictly teaching positions in medicine, but we actually had a faculty member who just supervised our resident ENT clinic. She had worked as a surgeon for years, but eventually gave up her surgical practice and worked part-time in our clinic.

Another way to change your practice is to consider locum tenens. This can be a temporary or a permanent choice. I talked about locum tenens in Section One, and have mixed feelings about it. I really enjoyed working in Alaska and Hawaii, and being able to work part-time. At some point, the quality of work done by my locums company really deteriorated, and I eventually got frustrated with how much money the company was earning off me. Since you never really know what's going to happen in life, it's good to keep this as an option. I don't know if any of the companies are superior to the rest, but you are allowed to work with multiple different companies, even at the same time.

If you're considering other fields in medicine, you might have to do another residency. Have at it if you want, but I don't think I could do it. If you don't want any clinical practice component, you may be able to branch out in research without additional training. You could also consider teaching at a university. Some colleges hire MDs in addition to PhDs. You're likely to take a drastic pay cut (being married to a professor, I am aware of the salary differences), but your schedule will improve significantly, as well.

Some people leave medicine completely and start a second career. This could be in finance, running a bed and breakfast, or becoming a travel writer. If you find that you're passionate about something, don't ignore that. It might be best to do it more as a hobby (especially if it is not financially feasible), at least for a time. Changing careers is a big decision, but it might be the best option if you are totally miserable in medicine. Also, you won't be as effective caring for your patients if your heart isn't in it. Your friends and family probably want you to be happy, too!

Chapter Two: Insurance

I volunteer with an organization called Junior Achievement (link in index, as it's a great way to get involved in your community!). Twice per year, we do an activity called Finance Park, where middle and high school students get practice in making a family budget. We discuss mortgages, car payments, groceries, educational debt, and much more. Several of the budget line-items are different types of insurances. Most of us are probably familiar with at least the concept of insurance – paying a small(er) amount to avoid paying a large amount for something you hope doesn't happen. However, how much do we actually know about each type of insurance? Hopefully you won't have to use these insurances much, but having appropriate insurance helps with peace of mind and family finances.

I'm not going in depth on all of the insurances available, only the ones I think you need to know most about as a physician. Vision and dental are pretty self-explanatory, and are often offered as employment benefits. Auto and home go hand-in-hand with the respective purchases. I do talk to the Junior Achievement students about state minimum versus comprehensive coverage and cash value versus replacement cost, so make sure you know about these if you're choosing among policies.

1. Health Insurance

I'll start with this, since you all know what it is. I'll focus on some concepts you might not be aware of, though. Currently, there is a financial penalty if you do NOT have health insurance. Before that started, there was a period of a couple months where I did not have health insurance between finishing my residency and starting my first job. I will tell you that I felt kind of nervous during this time. I was worried that something might happen and I would be stuck with a big bill. Not having health insurance is not a good feeling.

In truth, although I did not have health insurance, I could have gotten it retroactively through COBRA. COBRA stands for "Consolidated Omnibus Budget Reconciliation Act" (in case you were wondering). Basically, it allows you to keep your insurance for a limited time when you leave your job. COBRA is generally available from companies that employ more than 20 people and can last up to 18 months (according to the U.S. Department of Labor). The thing that seems strange to me about COBRA is that you don't have to opt in or out right away. Therefore, you can have it in your "mental back pocket" but avoid paying premiums unless you use it. There is a limited time (18 to 36 months) for which you can do this though, so make sure you're aware of the deadlines if you choose to do it this way. When you leave your employer, they should send you a packet about COBRA insurance. If you are considering using it, make sure you read the packet so you know how to do it right. The major downside is that COBRA insurance is very expensive if you end up purchasing it.

If you don't have the option of employer-sponsored health insurance, the health insurance marketplace (healthcare.gov) is usually a cheaper choice than COBRA. I ended up using the marketplace when I was taking time off between jobs a couple years ago. However, trying to use the website brought me to tears since I got so frustrated. I accidentally ended up applying for Medicaid and my husband had to take over. I'm really not that bad with computers, but that was an incredibly horribly designed website. Thankfully, if you are working for a hospital or group practice, you are likely to be offered employer-sponsored health insurance. This is usually heavily subsidized by your employer, so you only pay a small per cent of the premium. You can usually elect to cover your dependents, as well (often for a higher premium).

Make sure you read the options in choosing your plan. Most employers offer more than one option. If they have a high-deductible plan, this one generally has the lowest premiums. It may also have the option to combine with a health savings account (HSA). If you are healthy and do not expect to have many medical costs for a couple years, this may make a lot of sense. Some employers contribute money to the HSA for you, and you can also contribute pre-tax dollars into the HSA to pay for health-related expenses (doctor's visits, medications, contact lenses, etc). If you are in the plan for 1-2 years, you can easily have enough in your HSA to cover your deductible. Unlike a flexible spending account

(FSA), the HSA does NOT have to be used up each year. Also, you get to keep the account even if you change insurances. If you do NOT have a high-deductible plan, you are not allowed to contribute to an HSA. If you have an HSA from a prior plan, though, you can still use it to pay for eligible expenses. Financially, it makes sense to max out your HSA at least until you get a good amount of money in there. Since you get to keep it forever, and you will probably have health care costs at some time, it's nice to have that tax-free money available.

Even though it's not really health insurance, I'll explain the FSA now. FSA can be used for health care expenses – like the HSA – but it expires at the end of each year. Another common FSA-eligible (but NOT HSA-eligible) expense is child care costs. The FSA can be used for elder care costs, as well. FSA is a pre-tax account like the HSA. Basically, if you have known expenses that qualify to be covered by an FSA, it makes sense to use it since it has tax benefits. However, you do NOT want to have extra money in your FSA at the end of the year, because you lose whatever you do not spend. For example, if you know child care will cost you $500 each month and you are keeping your child there for the whole year, it makes sense to put $6000 ($500/month x 12 months) into the account. If you know that your prescription copays are $100/month, you can put $1200 into it. If you are planning to use an FSA, check your specific plan details to make sure you use the plan appropriately.

In choosing your health insurance plan, think about your dependents and projected health care costs for the year. Generally, more coverage costs more money. If you know you are going to be using it a lot, though, it might make sense to pay the higher premiums. Just make sure you actually read the plan to find out the details on what is covered/not covered, premiums, co-pays, co-insurance, deductibles, and participating doctors/hospitals (a.k.a. in network/out of network). Make sure you pay attention to annual enrollment/enrollment periods so you do not miss out on insurance benefits. Some plans will give you a discount or rebate for healthy choices and behaviors, so take advantage of these opportunities, too.

2. Life Insurance

When I ask the students what life insurance is, someone will usually say, "Somebody gets money if you die." This is a good basic summary. With the commonly known type of life insurance (term insurance), the insured individual names one or more beneficiaries. The insurance is for a certain dollar amount and covers the insured for a fixed period of time. When the insured individual dies, the beneficiary gets that dollar amount, as long as the premiums have been payed continuously. To get life insurance, you often have to go through a physical exam to determine how healthy you are. The healthiest people pay the lowest premiums (because you are less likely to die soon if you are healthy, so the insurance company makes a lower-risk "bet" on you). Some life insurance plans are available without an exam, but they usually come with higher premium costs and/or lower payouts. It's best to get a term life insurance policy when you are young and healthy, since you "lock-in" that rate when you purchase the plan.

So who needs life insurance, and how much do you need? If you are a single person, have no dependents, and have no debts, you probably don't really need life insurance. If you want to have it as a "legacy" where you want your niece (for example) to get money when you die, you could get insurance for that purpose. You could also do a small policy just to cover burial costs. More commonly, though, you want to have life insurance to cover costs your dependent survivors would incur when you're gone. If you have a spouse that stays home to take care of your 3 children and you are the only one who earns a paycheck, your family might really struggle if you suddenly die. This is especially true if you add in a mortgage and educational debt. So to determine the amount of coverage you need, add up your debts and how much money you think your family needs when you're gone. To figure out those exact numbers, you might want to ask a financial planner or do some online research. My husband and I don't have kids, and we each have jobs, so we chose to each have life insurance that covers a little more than the mortgage.

You are able to change your insurance amounts over time if you desire. If you want to reduce your coverage, you just contact the company and they take care of it. If you want to increase your coverage at a later date, you often have to do another physical exam. Also, if you don't pay your premium, your policy will end. So if you want to keep your life insurance, make sure you continue to pay your premiums.

A second type of life insurance is whole (or permanent) life insurance. This is really an investment option combined with an insurance policy, so we will discuss it in the financial planning section.

3. Disability Insurance

Disability insurance pays you a portion of your income (usually anywhere from 40% to 80%) if you are unable to work. Many employers offer disability insurance policies. Some give a small amount for free, so you might as well opt in to any free coverage. However, the policies employers offer for purchase are generally not what we really need as physicians. If you are interested in their offerings, definitely ask human resources at your job.

There are several different types of disability insurance. Disability insurance is often broken down into short-term and long-term disability. Short-term disability generally lasts up to 6 months, whereas long-term is anywhere from a year to life-time. There is a waiting period before disability benefits start, with 7-14 days for short-term and an average of 90 days for long-term. A brief but helpful link is given in the index for more information, and insurance agencies will be more than happy to give you information on their policies. Make sure you shop around to get the best plan for you. How much and what type(s) of disability insurance you choose to purchase depend on your financial needs and plans.

As opposed to a generic long-term disability policy, what most physicians want to purchase is a specialty-specific policy. This is especially true for surgeons. For example, if I lost my pinky or developed a mild tremor, a doctor performing a general disability exam might say that I am not disabled. However, if I have a specialty-specific policy that states my occupation as ENT surgeon, I could still earn disability benefits since either of those conditions would make me unlikely to be able to perform ENT surgery. If you have a policy like this, you can still earn disability benefits even if you can still perform a modified version of your job. In this situation, I might still choose to see patients in the clinic, but since I can no longer perform the same surgeries, I can get both my clinic income and disability income. This might sound unfair, but most of us surgeons go through the torment of surgical residency because surgery is our favorite part of the job. If we can no longer operate, that's a big loss.

You can search for disability policies on your own, or use a professional. I chose to get disability insurance while in my residency through a company that only works with physicians. They were able to show my husband and I different disability options. We made our own choices, but it was helpful to have them to tell us what was available.

Like life insurance, disability insurance usually involves a physical exam, so it's best to get this when you're young and healthy, too. If you buy them both at the same time, you may be able to just do 1 physical exam. Again, the insurance goes away if you don't pay your premiums, so make sure to pay your premiums if you want to keep the insurance. You can generally increase your disability insurance if your salary increases. There is usually not another exam in this case, but you have to show proof of income. Your premium will increase if you increase the coverage, but the payout increases, as well. There are usually limits to how often you can increase the coverage, so check this on your policy.

4. Malpractice Insurance

Yuck. We wish we didn't have to think about this, but it's a reality in American medicine. Thankfully, if you are an employed physician, your basic malpractice insurance should be covered. The most common limit I see is $1 million/$3 million. This means that the insurer would cover up to $1 million per claim and $3 million per year. For low-to-average risk specialties, I would think that this would be more than enough. For higher-risk fields (surgery and OB/GYN), some people choose to purchase their own personal malpractice to supplement their employer-sponsored policy. It is hard to know if you need to do this. There is a lot of variation from state-to-state as far as litigiousness, so you may want to ask your colleagues.

Your regular malpractice coverage is in effect only while you are working at your regular location. It often does not cover outside activities (moonlighting, mission work), so make sure you have coverage for those situations if applicable. Also, it generally does not cover fraud. So if you actively commit fraud, you will not be covered by your employer's policy. Please don't commit fraud anyways! It's horrible for the patients and the profession.

There's a lot more than can be said about malpractice insurance, but I think the last part you really need to know is tail coverage. When you leave a practice for any reason – getting a new job, retirement, career change – you need to make sure you have coverage for any claims that come up after you leave. This is called tail coverage. This was discussed in the Contracts chapter. As a reminder, make sure you know from your contract who is paying for what in this regard, as it could cost you upwards of $200,000 for the policy.

Chapter Three: Financial Planning

I already gave a disclaimer at the beginning of the book, but it bears repeating. All of the information in this book, and particularly the financial section, is based on my own experience and research. I am not a financial planner, lawyer, or magician. Please consult these professionals as needed, and make sure to do your own research. This information is provided as a starting point and does not substitute for professional guidance.

Do you want to worry about money? I don't know anyone who would say 'yes' to this question. As a physician, you are lucky enough to be in a profession where money is more readily available than many other careers. In the Finance Park exercise I mentioned above, we give students annual salaries from 30K to 90K. If you work full-time as any type of physician, you will earn more than this. All of the students end up being able to make the budgets work, even the ones with the lowest salaries. Since they are 8th graders and you have an advanced degree, you should be able to do it, too. Yes, you likely have student loans to pay off, but you're in much better shape than the majority of Americans. So you don't have to worry about how to earn money, but you can still struggle financially if you don't learn to manage your money.

Here are my top 4 guidelines for financial security (read on for more details):
1) If you can't afford it, don't buy it. This is very simple but many Americans ignore it.
2) Stock an emergency fund. This will help you avoid bad things like credit card debt and relying on payday loans.
3) Look at interest rates. You want to take advantage of interest rates that are favorable to you, and pay off debts with the highest interest rates first.
4) Save money and save money. The first one means to put money into savings (and investments), and the second means avoid spending money frivolously.

1. Saving

In a recent survey, 1/3 of Americans had absolutely no money saved, and another 1/3 had less than $1000 saved (link in index). I was pretty shocked the first time I heard this. Some people say, "Kim, it's easy for you to save money since you're a doctor." Well, I have been saving money since I got checks in my birthday cards from my grandparents as a kid. My husband and I contributed money each month to a savings account when we lived in Philadelphia on his $20K grad student stipend. I truly believe – and financial professionals agree – that saving money has much less to do with your overall income than with your priorities. The amount you can save is often limited by your income, but even people making low salaries can – and *should* – put money into savings.

If you're reading this in medical school or residency, you're in the lower income group. If you're reading it during practice, you're making a higher income. If you've already retired, hopefully you've done the right things along the way so you can enjoy your retirement. Whatever the case, with each paycheck, make sure you are putting some money into your savings. The easiest way to do this is having it set up as an automatic contribution from your bank account with your direct deposit each pay period. Do NOT wait until the end of the month and just save what you have left over. If you are someone who always has money left over, this strategy is OK, but many people try and fail at this method. When they have money, they spend it until it is gone, and then there is nothing left to put into savings.

So what if you feel you don't have any money to put into your savings? It's very likely that you can make some cutbacks. In medical school, my husband and I didn't have much money. This was around the time where cell phones were getting more popular, but nowhere like they are now. We saved money by not having a land line (common now, but no so much then) and just having 1 cell phone for the two of us (seems almost implausible now, but seriously, people – you are WAY too addicted to your smartphones). Also, we did not have cable and just had an antenna for local TV stations. This was before online Netflix and Hulu and all the other streaming services. It was only 2005, but things have changed a lot since then! I also cooked most of the time, and we took leftovers for lunch (we still do this!). My husband made coffee at home and took it with him rather than buying Starbucks every day. We once had a dinner-and-a- movie date for $5 total (dollar theater and Fazoli's all-you-can-eat breadsticks). That was in 2001, but you can still find deals out there.

I didn't feel like I was being deprived, but this can be an issue for some people. If you don't like the idea of cutting your spending, think of it as a game – How much can we save this week? Or this month? Then try to beat it next time. Or just keep in mind how saving money along the weeks and years will let you retire while you're young enough to still enjoy it. Once you have a larger income and your savings are on track, you can choose to spend money on more luxury items. We have cable now. We like to go on trips. They used to be limited to driving or camping trips (which we still do), but now they can be international flights or cruises if we choose.

So how much should you save? Everyone has different advice, but we tell students in Junior Achievement to save 5-15% of their net monthly income. Another common goal is at least 10%. You might be on the lower side of this in medical school or residency, but can probably easily exceed this when you are an attending. Again, when you are making a low income, the point is to get in the habit of saving. Also, the earlier you start saving, the longer you have compound interest working for you. Compound interest almost seems like magic. The money you earn on the money you save then goes on to earn you extra money. How great is that?

You should have 3 or 4 designated savings accounts. Some of these can be combined into the same bank account, but you should know how much money you have in each. The largest account (at least over time) should be your retirement account. People used to say you needed to have $1 million saved to retire, but that number is generally considered quite low now. The link in the index is an article that gives you tips on how to calculate how much you need to retire. Basically, it depends on how much money you can live on per year and how many years you plan to live after you retire (since we all know the answer to that question...). Many retirement accounts are tied up in plans that you cannot access without penalty until you reach a certain age. Therefore, you need to have funds in other accounts, as well. If you plan to retire early, you will need more in these other accounts.

So in addition to your retirement account, you will want to have a general savings account. Some of this may be your early retirement money, but you also need money that is accessible to pay bills each month. You may also have an account where you save for particular items, like a family vacation or a new car. (Note: I have never had a car payment. I have always saved up enough money to buy a car, then bought the car outright. This is easier with used cars, but gently used cars are generally a better deal than brand new cars because of the depreciation that happens as soon as you drive a new car off the lot. Saving up to buy a car makes a lot of sense if you can do it to avoid the interest payments.)

The final savings account you really need is an emergency fund. I had always heard the rule of thumb that you should have 3 months worth of expenses in an emergency fund. This idea behind this is that it takes an average of 3 months to find a new job. If you lose or quit your job, you still need to pay your bills. This is what the emergency fund is for. The nice thing about the emergency fund is that you don't have to keep contributing to it. Once you've saved the required amount, you just keep it there. You only have to add to it if you've used part of it. Some people say that you should have significantly more than this in an emergency fund – even as much as a year's worth of expenses. I don't know who's right, but 3 months is a lot better than nothing. If you don't have this emergency fund, you may turn to less financially sound options, like credit cards or payday loans. You could even lose your house or car. So fund your emergency fund as soon as possible!

2. Budgeting

If you are a very frugal person with a high income, you probably don't need to make a budget. Even in this case, though, it's a good idea to know where your money is going each month. Most

Americans just spend all the money that comes in, not really thinking about where it's going or why they're spending it. We'll go over how to make and adjust a budget.

A budget is usually done on a monthly basis. If you have a steady salary, you first want to calculate your net monthly income. You can start by combining two 2-week pay periods, or you can divide your annual income by 12. These numbers should be relatively close to each other. Then you need to subtract taxes. The federal rate ranges from 0% to 40% depending on salary. Once you are an attending, you will likely be in the 33-40% bracket. You'll also have to pay Medicare tax, and most states have a state tax rate, as well. So altogether, taxes will probably take out 40-50% of your gross pay. What is left is your net monthly income, which is the money you actually have available for savings, bills, and luxury items.

Let's go over the typical items in a budget, in approximate descending order of cost as percentage of your net monthly income.

Housing: Often 20-25%. May change based on local cost-of-living, but try not to overburden your budget with more house than you can afford.
Childcare: Depends on number and age of children, but can be up to 15%
Savings: Numbers vary, but try to save at least 10%. If you have money left over in the budget, try to increase this.
Food: 10-15% (lower if you cook yourself, higher for dining out)
Transportation: 5-10% (includes car payment, gas, maintenance)
Insurances: 10-15% (health, disability, life, home, auto)
Educational debt: 2-10%
Credit card debt: hopefully 0, but could be much higher
Health care: 5-10% (out-of-pocket expenses)
Utilities: around 5%
Philanthropy/charitable giving: 0-10%
Recreation/fun money: depends (see below)

If you search the internet, you will see many different numbers. One common suggestion is the 50/20/30 rule, where 50% of the budget goes to needs (housing, transportation, childcare, food, insurances, utilities), 20% goes to savings and debt, and 30% goes towards your wants. Spending a whopping 30% of your budget on wants seems pretty irresponsible to me. I guess if you can cover everything else with the 70%, that is OK. However, some of that 30% may go toward the bigger house or nicer car, which are things you don't really need.

There are a number of online tools and apps available to help you make a budget. I have listed one in the index, but have not personally used it myself. You can also sit down with pencil and paper and figure it out. I recommend making a plan first, where you take your income and put a proposed dollar amount on each line item. At the end of the month, see how much you actually spent on each item. Don't forget to add in the monthly average for bills like insurance payments that only come 1-4 times per year. If you find you have spent more than you budgeted in a certain category, see where you have some money left over and figure out where you need to save money. If you're considering buying a new house, see how much you can actually afford for your monthly payment rather than just buying the most expensive house for which you are approved.

What if you have extra money in your budget after you've accounted for your savings, debts, and needs? This is a great situation, and will probably be the case for most attendings. First, it is OK to put some money towards wants. Part of the reason we put in all the time and effort to become a doctor is to be able to enjoy our lives. However, I strongly recommend against spending significant money on luxury items until you have yourself in good financial shape. Before contributing a lot to "fun money," I would do the following:

1) Make sure you have an emergency fund (at least 3 months of expenses).
2) Make sure you have zero credit card debt. Credit cards are usually charging you 16-18% interest on your balance if you don't pay them off each month. Some even charge up to 30%. There is virtually NO long-term investment that can given you this rate of

return on a consistent basis. So having credit card debt when you are able to pay it off is basically throwing money away.

3) Make sure you are where you should be as far as saving for retirement. You can use the retirement calculator in the index, your own research, or a financial planner.

You can always add leftover money to your savings/investments. It just makes that next trip or retirement even closer! There are many charities that would love to help you in your conundrum, too. Remember that philanthropy is tax deductible. You will have to pay back all of your loans at some point, so you can contribute extra here, as well. Just make sure you're considering interest rates (see below).

3. Debt

Almost all of us have debt when we start our professional lives. The average is around $200,000 for physicians right out of medical school. Yes, you do have to pay it back eventually, but it is helpful to think of good debt versus bad debt.

Educational debt is usually considered good debt. You are making the choice to go into debt to invest in yourself and your future. Many studies have shown that people with education beyond high school make much more on average than those who stop with a high school diploma. Although you have to go into debt to start, you should be able to pay it off with your improved future earnings. Most of us don't have 200K just sitting around at age 18, so we don't have much of a choice with it. There are a few schools that have free tuition for their medical students, but this isn't very common. I paid off my educational debt within 3 years of finishing residency, and even my less frugal friend just told me she paid hers off within the same period (and she even did a fellowship after residency). So as long as you are working as a physician and making sound financial decisions, you really shouldn't have to worry about paying off this debt.

The second type of good debt is a mortgage. With a mortgage rather than rent, you are buying equity in a home. As long as you make your payments, you will eventually own the home. Your home becomes an asset (rather than a debt) as soon as the remaining mortgage is less than 50% of the appraised value of the home, which is much sooner than the end of the loan in most cases. Also, paying the mortgage payments on time each month helps your credit score. (This is actually true of any debt payments you make on time.) Buying a home may not be financially possible based on your current finances or geographic location, but it usually a sound financial decision if you can do it. Also, if the mortgage rates are very low, taking out a mortgage can actually be a good investment strategy. When we bought our most recent home, mortgage rates were below 3%. With the stock market averaging returns of 8-12% over the last several decades, it made sense to take out the mortgage at 3% and leave the cost of the house invested in the stock market. (By the way, mortgage rates and bank interest rates are tied to the prime rate or "prime lending rate." This is an interesting concept I encourage you to investigate if you like this sort of thing. It helps make interest rates make more sense.)

So what is bad debt? Probably the worst one is credit card debt. Credit cards can be a great tool, but you have to use them wisely. My husband and I buy almost everything with credit cards, because we have credit cards that give us cash back. The KEY to making this work is to make sure you pay off your bill in full at the end of each month. If you don't pay it off, you end up paying much more than the face value of your purchase, and it can be hard to climb out of the hole. Back to financial recommendation #1: If you can't afford it, don't buy it! When it comes to emergency situations, hopefully you can use your emergency fund or other resources. Just for clarification, an emergency is not, "This Gucci purse will only be on sale for 2 more days!" An emergency is, "My son just broke his leg and needs to have surgery." If your only option seems to be using a credit card, make sure to pay it off as soon as possible. In Finance Park, we show the students that the average American household credit card debt is over $15,000. This is shocking to me. I wish everyone could go through Finance Park or read this book to try to avoid that from happening!

Another type of bad debt is the payday loan. Basically, you go to a lender and get an advance on your next paycheck. A typical situation may be that they give you $100 two weeks before you get your paycheck, and you have to pay them back the $100 plus a $15 to $40 fee once the pay check arrives. This is $40 that could have been in your own pocket if you had budgeted your money properly for the month, or had money you could have used in your emergency fund. Payday loans are convenient, but they are definitely a bad financial strategy – well, for everyone except the lender.

So if you have multiple debts, which should you pay off first? Most will have a minimum monthly payment. Make sure you pay at least this much each month. An easy way to pay things off faster is to round up. If your minimum payment on one of your educational loans is $189.26, just go ahead and pay $200 each month. You probably won't miss that extra $10.74, and you will pay off your loan faster. The smartest way to choose which ones to overpay is to look at the interest rates. Beyond the minimum payments, divert any extra money to the ones with the highest interest rates. This saves you the most money over time. Education loans tend to have relatively low interest rates in general, and many have provisions that serially lower the interest rates with continued on-time payments. By the time I finished paying off my student loans, the interest rate was down to less than 0.5%. If interest rates on your loans are very low, you may want to just make the minimum payments and invest any extra money as you will likely earn more in the market.

4. Investing

We talked earlier about how important saving is. However, if you just put your money in a bank account, it will actually lose value over time due to inflation. With the prime rate being low, bank savings account rates are very low, too, so your money sitting in the bank earns you a pitiful amount of interest. To grow your wealth, you will generally need to invest your money. Remember, this is just my own strategy. Make sure to do your own research and consult financial professionals liberally.

When starting off with investing, people break investments into low risk and high risk. Low risk investments have a very small chance of losing your money. The main advantage of low risk investments is that you don't have to worry (much) about losing your money. However, your return on these investments is relatively low, as well. Higher risk investments are ones where you risk losing some or all of your investment, but you generally get a much higher return on your investment. The high risk investment we will discuss is the stock market. There are always "trends" that come up and smaller niches – "bitcoin," gold, real estate – but we won't cover those here. There are plenty of websites and financial advisors who can help you with that. Make sure to watch out for con artists, though!

Each person should have a diversified investment portfolio. This is a fancy way of saying, "Don't put all your eggs in one basket." You should have some combination of lower risk/lower return products and higher risk/higher return products. Generally, the younger you are, the more high risk your portfolio can be. This is because if something bad happens, you have time to make the money back. If you are getting close to retirement age, you generally want a lower overall risk. If all your money is in stocks and the market crashes just as you go to retire, you can be in trouble.

There are several low risk options. The first is a CD, or certificate of deposit. You buy a CD (usually through a bank) for a certain dollar amount, and agree to leave your money there for a certain amount of time (generally a few months to a few years). For lending them your money for this time, you get a small fee as an interest rate. The rates are better for you when the prime rate is high, so they're not so great right now. Government bonds and corporate bonds from large, stable companies are also considered low risk in general. Individual bonds can sometimes be several thousand dollars, so you can also buy a bond index fund (see below for more information on index funds). Most people think the US government will not go out of business, so is unlikely to default on its bonds. If a company goes out of business, the bondholders get paid before the stockholders, but it's still possible to lose money.

Another low-risk option is whole life insurance. This is also known as permanent or universal life insurance. Large companies often use this, but it didn't seem very useful to my husband and I when a financial planner was recommending it to us. With whole life insurance, there is a death benefit like in term life. However, the premiums are much higher because you are basically paying into an account that builds cash value. This account can earn interest, is tax-deferred, and you can borrow from it. You have to pay into it for many years or over pay early on to get much of a return, though, and the return rates tend to be much lower than the stock market. If you are interested, look into it, but make sure you know what you are getting into.

So what's the best investment strategy for the stock market? Talk to 20 people, and you'll hear 20 opinions. We all hear about ups and downs of the stock market. Some people made a fortune buying Apple at the right time, and others have lost everything. It's unlikely that you'll hit on the next Apple. Historically, the investors who have done the best over time are generally those who keep their money in the market and continue to buy stocks irregardless of the what the market is doing. This sounds scary, but numbers over time support it.

There are a multiple ways to invest in the stock market. You can hire someone to do it for you. You will usually give them some direction, as far as if you want to concentrate on certain industries and how risky you want the portfolio to be, but they will do the leg work. On the opposite side of the spectrum, you can choose each individual stock you want to buy. There is generally a fee for purchasing the stock, but there are plenty of online sites that allow you to do this (e-trade, Fidelity, Vanguard, etc). Buying individual stocks is probably the riskiest option (unless you are illegally doing it through insider trading or you have an awesome *Back to the Future* flux capacitor method of predicting the future). You essentially lose all the money invested in that stock if the company goes bankrupt or does poorly.

Instead of buying individual stocks, many investors buy small amounts of multiple companies. The most well-known example of this is the mutual fund. Mutual funds have been around for 100+ years. They can be actively or passively managed. An actively managed mutual fund is a group of stocks that has been selected by an individual who supposedly has some knowledge of the market. There are also passively managed mutual funds that track an index like the S&P 500. Some are intentionally designed as low risk vs. high risk, or may be focused in a single industry (e.g. health care or technology). There is a management fee for each mutual fund, and the minimum purchase amount is often several thousand dollars. Each fund has a prospectus that shows how the fund has done over time, but no one can really predict how it will do over the future.

Since the stock market as a whole tends to grow over time, things called index funds have also been created. Instead of having someone choose individual stocks as in an actively managed mutual fund, an index fund takes a large collection of stocks like the S&P 500 or Russell 2000. The stocks are represented in the index fund in the same proportion as they are in the stock market (i.e. you get a bigger "piece" of a bigger company and a smaller piece of a small company). Since there is no individual changing what stocks or ratio of stocks go into the index, the index funds are considered to be "passively managed." This generally equates to lower fees than mutual funds. Also, since we talked about the fact that the market as a whole tends to grow over time, this is a way of taking advantage of that overall growth.

A variation of index funds that has come about in the past 30 years is the exchange-traded fund (ETF). ETFs essentially allow you to buy shares of an index fund through the stock market. Management fees are generally lower, and there may or may not be a fee to purchase the fund itself. It is free to purchase Vanguard ETFs through a Vanguard account, or Fidelity ETFs through a Fidelity account. Minimum purchase amounts are often much less than mutual funds, at about $100 rather than several thousand dollars. One of the most seemingly logical ways to take advantage of the stock market is buying small amounts of multiple companies, and ETFs allow you to do that.

Many employers will have some sort of investment fund as one of their employee benefits. These usually come with tax advantages, and are generally known as 401(k) plans (or 403(b) for nonprofit organizations). You can usually choose to contribute some part of your salary, which is put into the fund before taxes. This allows you to avoid paying taxes on the portion of your salary that was put into the fund. You instead pay the taxes when you withdraw the money later on. Most of us physicians will be in a higher tax bracket when we are earning our regular pay than we will be when we go to withdraw the money upon retirement, so it ends up saving money in taxes. There is a limit on how much you can put into a 401(k), but it is usually wise to contribute up to the limit if you can afford it.

There is an opposite tax deferral method for people who earn a lower income now than they expect to earn in the future. This is a Roth IRA. Some employers offer Roth 403(b) accounts and Roth 401(k) accounts, too. The IRA part just means "individual retirement account." IRAs are individual savings plans with tax benefits that generally have defined annual contribution limits and assess a penalty if you take your money out prior to retirement age. The Roth IRA is available to individuals who make LESS than a certain amount (which changes year to year). It allows you to pay taxes when you put the money into an account, but you don't have to pay taxes when you withdraw the money. This is a good option for the students and residents out there before you start making the big bucks.

Some employers also offer contribution matching as a benefit. Find out if your employer does this, and make sure you take advantage of it. It is free money! You often have to work there for 6-12 months before the benefit starts, and you sometimes have to stay several years for it to be fully "vested." This means that if you leave before that time period, you don't get to keep some or all of the money the employer contributed. (You won't lose your contributions, though.) What happens with the match is that if you put some of your paycheck into the account, the employer will contribute extra money into the account. For example, in my residency, my employer matched 50% of my contribution up to 4% of my total salary. This means that when I put 4% of my salary into the retirement account, my employer put an additional 2% of my salary into the account for me. This is like getting a 2% raise just for saving money. They are generally smart enough to cap it at some low number, so you can't save 50% of your paycheck and get them to give you a 25% bonus. That would be nice.

IRAs are advisable due to the tax benefits, and employer matches are good since they're free money. You will have other retirement accounts, as well, since there are contribution limits on these special ones. With any retirement account or other financial product through an employer, you usually are able to invest that money in a variety of ways. You may be limited to a single company (e.g. Fidelity) or have more freedom. Just make sure you know where your money is and what it's doing so it can work for you. You worked hard for it in the first place!

Conclusion

I truly hope this book will be helpful to you. I really enjoyed writing parts of it, while others were more of a struggle. We all made it, though (even if you just skipped to the end!). Please use the information in the text and the index as jumping-off points to help you learn more about these topics. Best wishes for a happy, productive life and career!

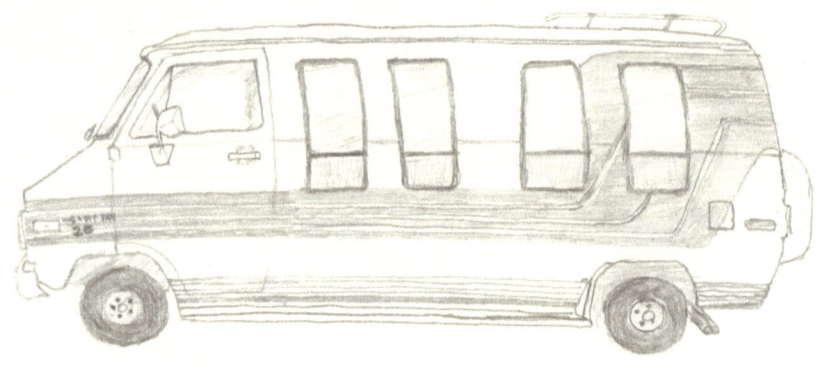

Our camping van, as sketched by my husband
A source of much enjoyment!

Appendix 1: Website Links

SECTION ONE
U.S. News & World Report
- Annual rankings of medical schools for research and primary care
http://grad-schools.usnews.rankingsandreviews.com/best-graduate-schools/top-medical-schools

Association of American Medical Colleges (AAMC)
- All recognized medical schools with links to individual school web pages
https://members.aamc.org/eweb/DynamicPage.aspx?site=AAMC&webcode=AAMCOrgSearchResult&orgtype=Medical%20School
- Tables with extensive data on applicants, matriculants, graduates, and more
https://www.aamc.org/data/facts/
- List of all residencies and fellowships participating in ERAS ("The Match")
https://services.aamc.org/eras/erasstats/par/index.cfm

Medscape (may need to login)
- Physician compensation report for 2019
https://www.medscape.com/slideshow/2019-compensation-overview-6011286

American Medical Association (AMA)
- Resources for how to choose a specialty (better access if you are a member)
https://www.ama-assn.org/residents-students/career-planning-resource/choosing-medical-specialty

Doximity
- Residency Navigator program that allows you to compare residencies
https://residency.doximity.com/

Accreditation Council for Graduate Medical Education (ACGME)
- Page to check accreditation by program
https://apps.acgme.org/ads/Public/Programs/Search

Big Interview
- List of questions during interviews with additional interviewing tips
http://biginterview.com/blog/2014/09/residency-interview-questions.html

Mindful Surgeon
- Blog by one of my colleagues that focuses on physician wellness and career navigation; link directly to the article I wrote on locum tenens
http://mindfulsurgeon.com/2019/05/01/off-the-beaten-path-the-locum-tenens-option-for-a-surgeon/

SECTION TWO

FVCS FAQs
- Includes list of states which require FCVS
https://www.fsmb.org/licensure/fcvs/fcvs_faq

Medically Underserved Areas
- Allows you to lookup official designation of areas within the US
https://data.hrsa.gov/

Medical job search sites
- not an exhaustive listing by any means, but includes some of the most popular
www.practicelink.com
www.practicematch.com
www.mdjobsite.com
www.nejmcareercenter.org
https://careers.jamanetwork.com/

SECTION THREE

Physician Fee Schedule Search
- searchable tool that provides global period and RVU values for each CPT code
- you must agree to the search terms, but it is free
https://www.cms.gov/apps/physician-fee-schedule/license-agreement.aspx

Time-Based Coding Guidelines
- helpful table from AAFP that tells you the time requirements for different LOS codes (need to subscribe to use)
https://www.aafp.org/fpm/2003/0600/fpm20030600p27-rt1.pdf

CMS 1995 Documentation Guidelines
https://www.cms.gov/Outreach-and-Education/Medicare-Learning-Network-MLN/MLNEdWebGuide/Downloads/95Docguidelines.pdf

CMS 1997 Documentation Guidelines
https://www.cms.gov/Outreach-and-Education/Medicare-Learning-Network-MLN/MLNEdWebGuide/Downloads/97Docguidelines.pdf

E/M University
– coding website; both free information and subscription services
– hover over gray boxes on left; good sub-menus with history, exam, and MDM information
– They do use the descriptive words from CMS that I find to be confusing rather than instructive, but there is still useful information here.
https://emuniversity.com/

Link to MDM table I created (small version also in Appendix 3):
https://drive.google.com/open?id=1mBCOiFITXLS5WCHv0oRdFtJI0flBiwQH

SECTION FOUR

Wikipedia city information
(https://en.wikipedia.org/wiki/
List_of_United_States_cities_by_population)

AMA Physician Lawsuit Article
https://wire.ama-assn.org/practice-management/1-3-physicians-has-been-sued-age-55-1-2-hit-suit
Harvard study on optimism and mortality
https://news.harvard.edu/gazette/story/2016/12/optistic-women-live-longer-are-healthier/

Junior Achievement: International organization that teaches financial literacy and job readiness in the modern world
https://www.juniorachievement.org/web/ja-usa/home

Additional information about short-term and long-term disability
https://www.policygenius.com/disability-insurance/short-term-disability-vs-long-term-disability-insurance/

Savings survey results
https://www.cnbc.com/2017/06/19/heres-how-many-americans-have-nothing-at-all-in-savings.html

Retirement calculator
https://www.cnbc.com/2018/04/11/how-to-figure-out-how-much-money-you-need-to-retire.html

Money Under 30: Site with lots of financial information geared at individuals under age 30
https://www.moneyunder30.com/

Budgeting site
https://www.everydollar.com/blog/budget-percentages

Appendix 2: Additional books you might find helpful
These are all available on Amazon.com

Communication in Medicine: A guide for students and physicians on interacting with patients, colleagues, and everyone else by Kimberly J. Kinder, MD

The Ultimate Guide to Choosing a Medical Specialty by Brian Freeman, MD
- has approximately 10- to 20-page discussions of each of 20 of the most common specialties

Learned Optimism by Martin E.P. Seligman

Feeling Good by David D. Burns

A PhD is Not Enough by physicist Peter J. Feibelman

Getting What You Came For by Robert L. Peters – advice on graduate school (recommended by my physicist husband)

Appendix 3: EMR help

EMR shortcut examples

New patient adult office visit (.npa for new patient adult)
- has entire template with HPI, ROS, History, Exam, A/P

Single words or phrases
.cho for cholesteatoma, .vs for vestibular schwannoma

Sentences or paragraphs
.srthy for surgical risks thyroidectomy
.pitin for patient info tinnitus

Exam template:
@Vs@ [pulls in vital signs]
The following areas were examined and were normal except as noted below:
Constitutional: General appearance of patient, assessment of ability to communicate and quality of voice
Head and Face: Inspection of overall appearance, palpation of sinuses for tenderness,
examination of salivary glands, assessment of facial strength
Eyes: ocular motility, general appearance
Ears: Otoscopic examination of external auditory canals and tympanic membranes, pneumo-otoscopy/TM mobility, assessment of hearing, external inspection of ears
Nose: Inspection of external nose, nasal mucosa, septum and turbinates
Oral cavity/Oropharynx: Inspection of lips, teeth, gums, oral mucosa, hard & soft palates, tongue, tonsils and posterior pharynx
Mirror: Inspection of larynx, hypopharynx, oropharynx, and nasopharynx
Neck: inspection and palpation of neck and thyroid
Respiratory: inspection of chest/work of breathing
Cardiovascular: palpation of temporal pulses
Lymphatic: palpation of neck nodes
Neurologic: evaluation of cranial nerves
Abnormalities/Comments: ***.

MDM Worksheet

For full size, go to following link:

https://drive.google.com/open?id=1mBCOiFITXLS5WCHv0oRdFtJI0flBiwQH

Smaller version on next page

A) Diagnoses	B) Data	C) Risk			
Add up points:	Add up points:	Highest value of ANY single item[3]:			
Self-limited/ minor: 1 pt[1]	Review/order lab test: 1 pt	≥1 chronic illness with severe exacerbation, progression, or treatment side effect Acute or chronic illness or injury that poses threat to life or bodily function (multiple trauma, MI, PE, ARF, psychiatric emergency) Abrupt change in neurologic status (e.g. seizure, TIA, weakness)	Cardiovascular imaging studies with contrast with risk factors Cardiac electrophysiology tests Diagnostic endoscopies with risk factors Discography	Elective major surgery with risk factors IV controlled substances Drug therapy requiring intensive monitoring for toxicity Decision not to resuscitate or to de-escalate care because of poor prognosis	4
Established problem, stable or improving: 1 pt	Review/order radiology test: 1 pt	≥1 chronic illness with mild exacerbation, progression, or treatment side effect ≥2 stable chronic illnesses Undiagnosed new problem with uncertain prognosis (e.g. lump in breast)	Physiologic tests under stress (cardiac stress test, fetal contraction stress test) Diagnostic endoscopies without risk factors Deep needle or incisional biopsy	Minor surgery with risk factors Elective major surgery without risk factors Prescription drug management Therapeutic nuclear medicine	3
Established problem, worsening or requiring additional intervention: 2 pt	Review/order medicine test (EKG, EEG, audiogram, PFT): 1 pt	Acute illness with systemic symptoms (e.g. colitis, pneumonitis) Acute complicated injury (e.g. head injury with brief LOC)	Cardiovascular imaging studies with contrast but without risk factors (arteriogram, cath) Obtain fluid from body cavity (e.g. lumbar puncture, thoracentesis)	IV fluids with additives Closed treatment of fracture or dislocation without manipulation	
New problem, no additional workup: 3 pt[2]	Discuss test with performing MD: 1 pt	≥2 self-limited/minor problems One stable chronic illness Acute uncomplicated illness or injury (e.g. allergies, sprain)	Physiologic tests not under stress (e.g. PFTs) Non-cardiovascular imaging studies with contrast (e.g. barium enema) Superficial needle biopsies Lab test requiring arterial puncture Skin biopsy	OTC drug management Minor surgery with no identified risk factors PT/OT IV fluids without additives	2
New problem with additional workup: 4 pt	Review and summation of old records or obtaining hx from person other than patient: 2 pt	One self-limited/minor problem	Test requiring venipuncture CXR EKG/EEG Urinalysis Ultrasound/echo KOH prep	Rest Gargles Elastic bandage Superficial dressing	1
	Decision to obtain old records: 1 pt				
	Independent review of image/tracing/ specimen: 2 pt				

Notes:
[1] maximum of 2 points for self-limited/minor diagnoses
[2] can only count 1 problem in this category per encounter (3 pts total)
[3] Reminder: Do not add points in Risk category. Just choose the single item in the table with the highest value.